Neurofibromatosis - Current Trends and Future Directions

Edited by Francesco Signorelli and Raffaella Messina

Published in London, United Kingdom

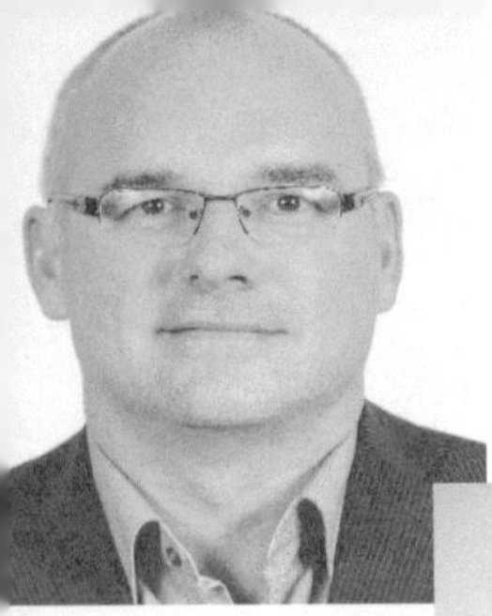
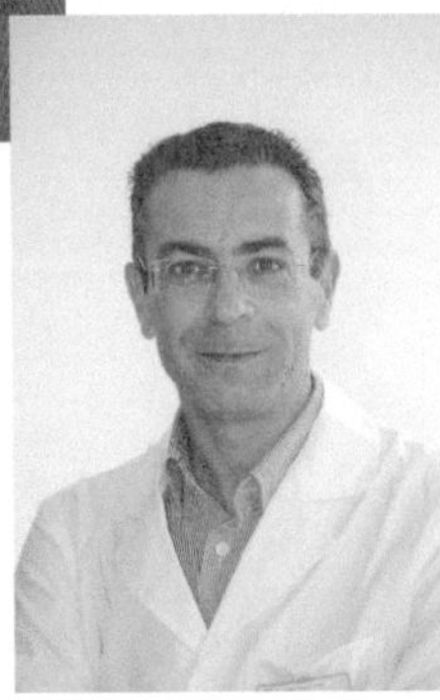
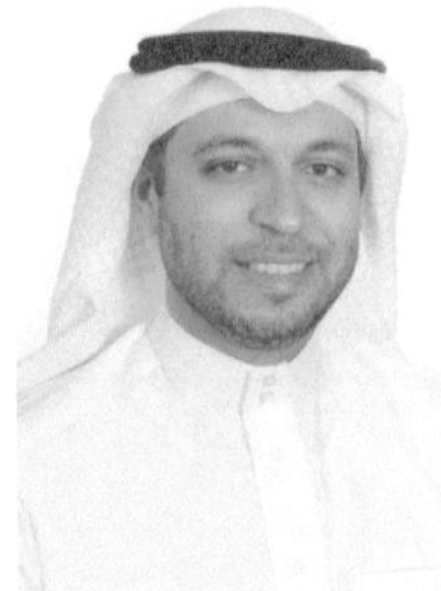
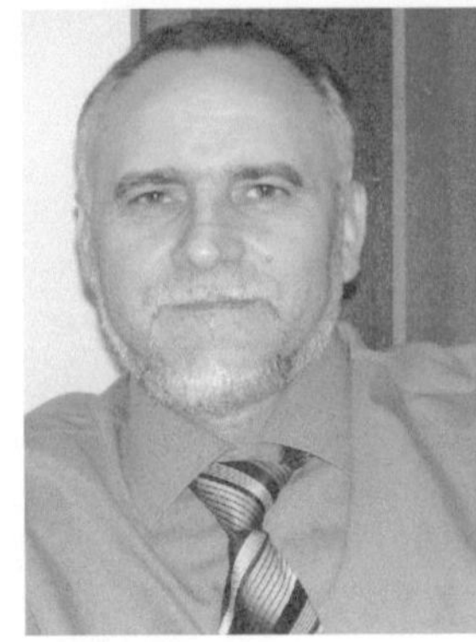
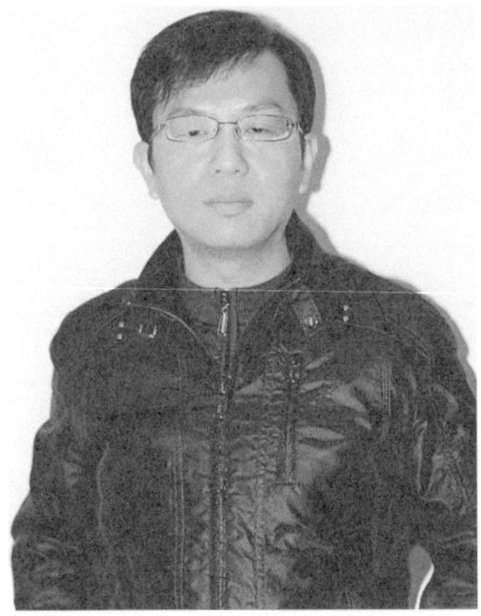
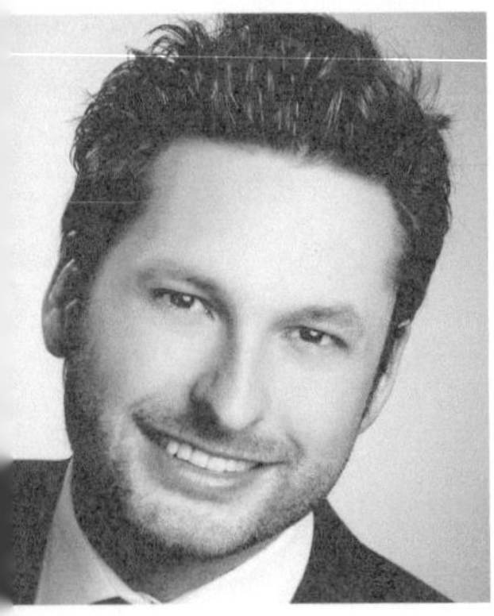
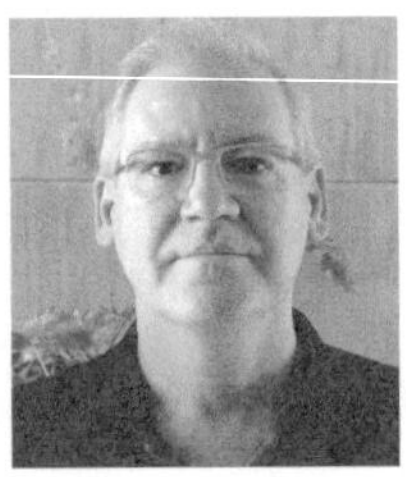

IntechOpen

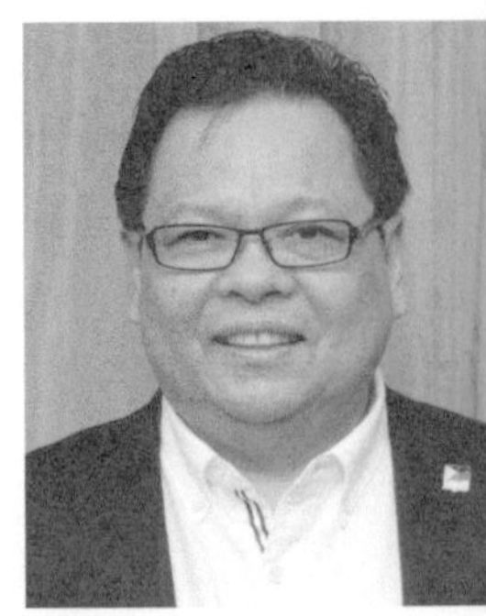
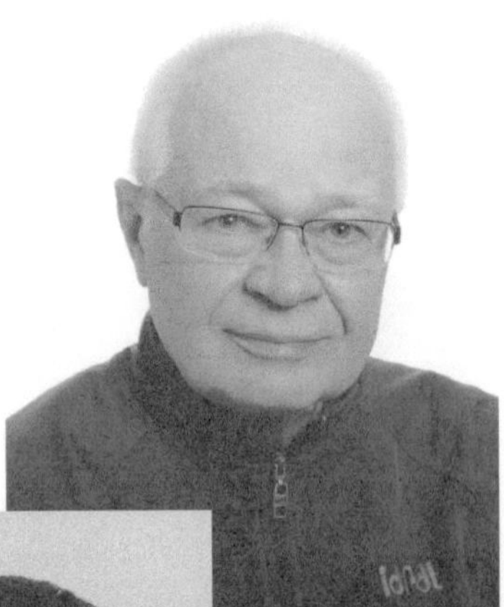
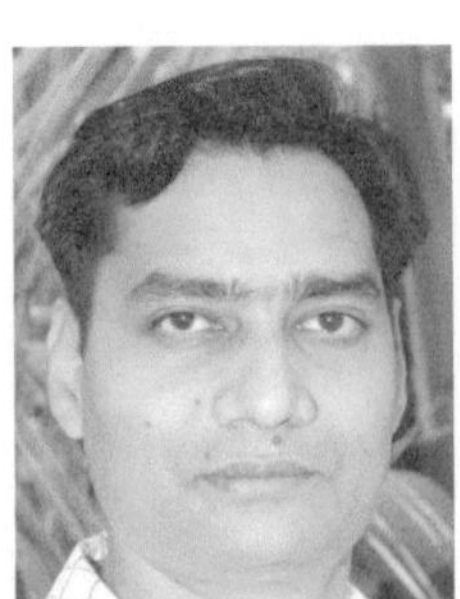
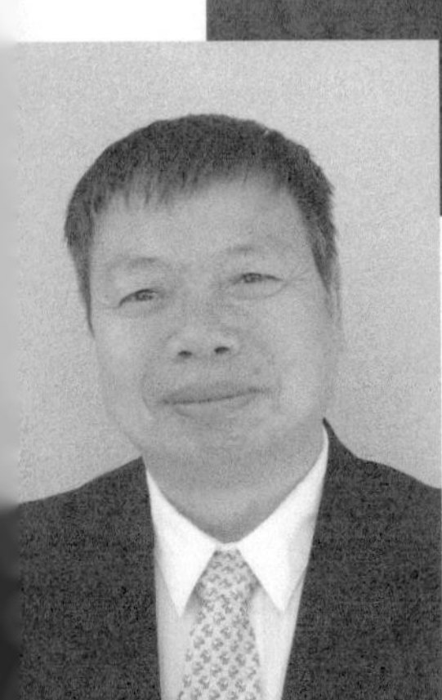
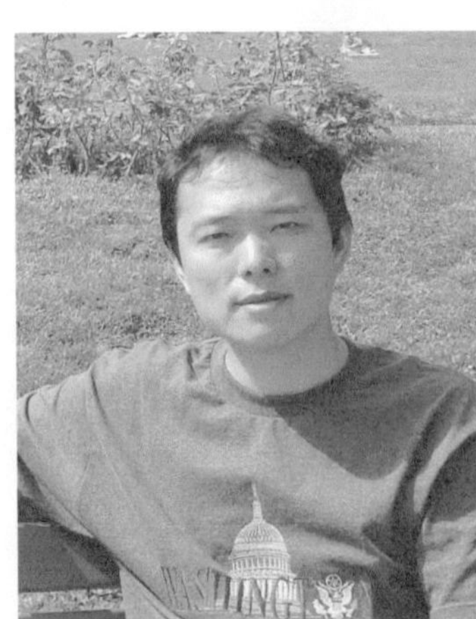
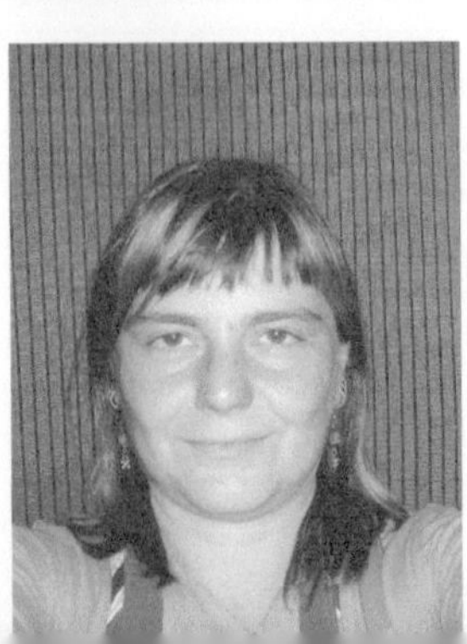

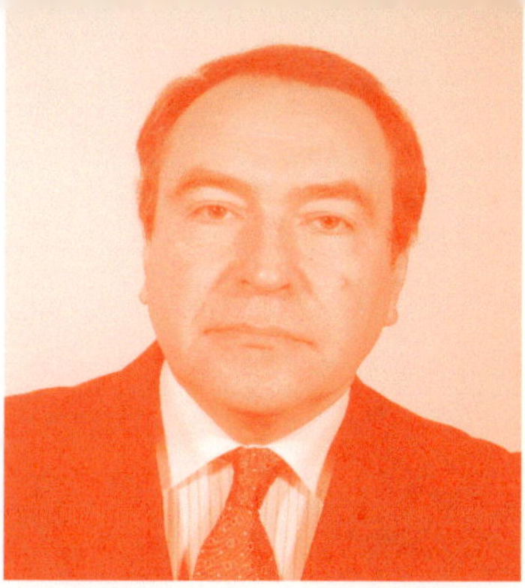
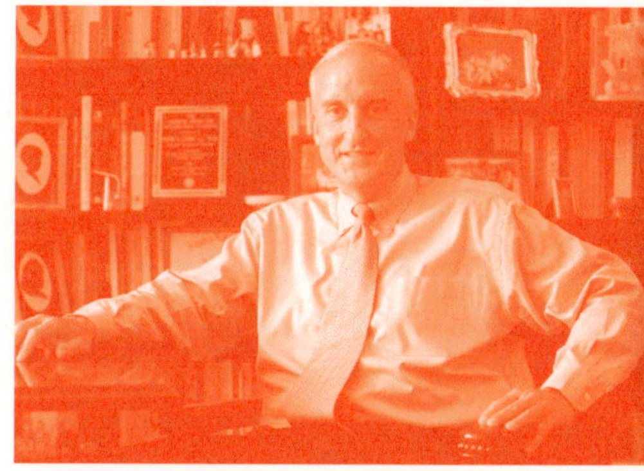
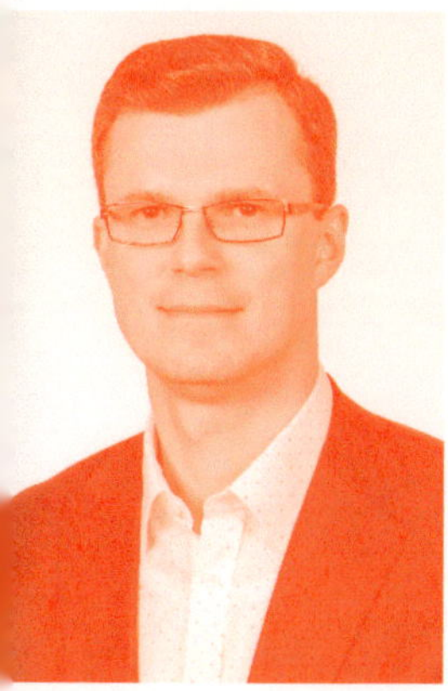
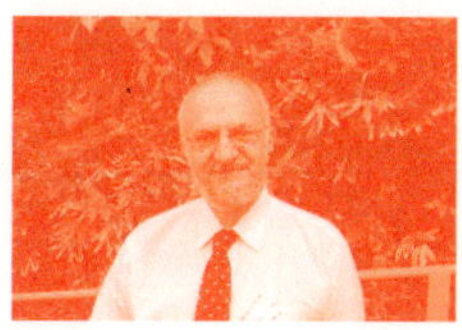
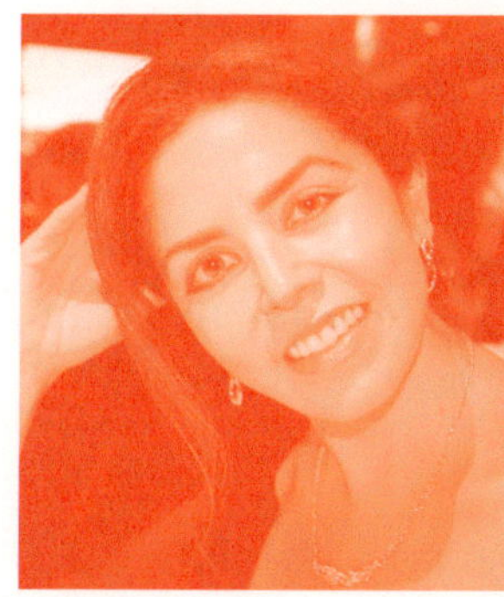

Supporting open minds since 2005

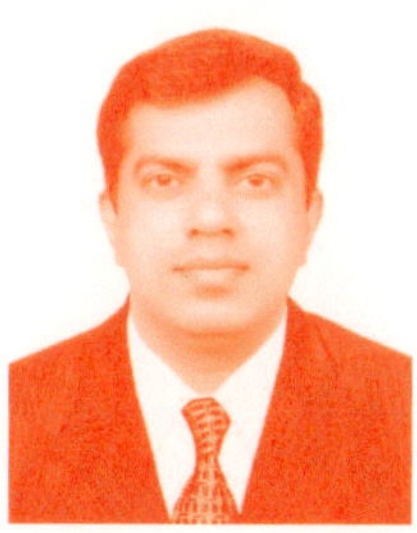
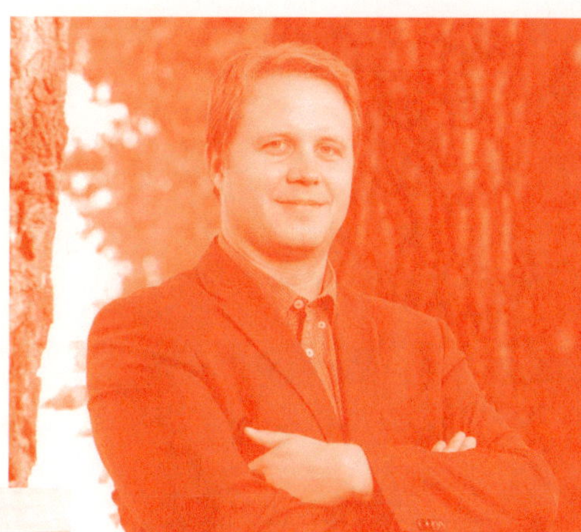
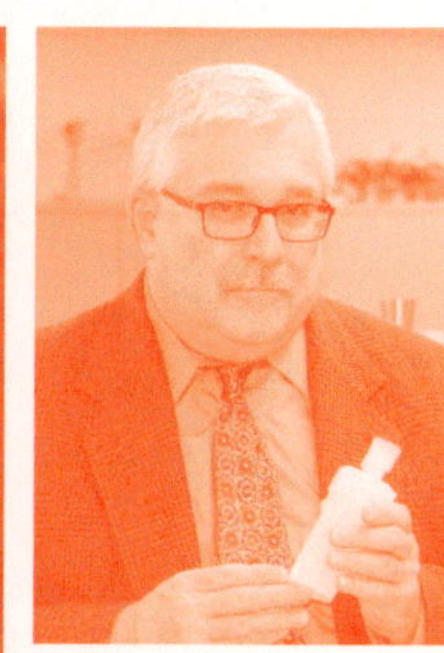
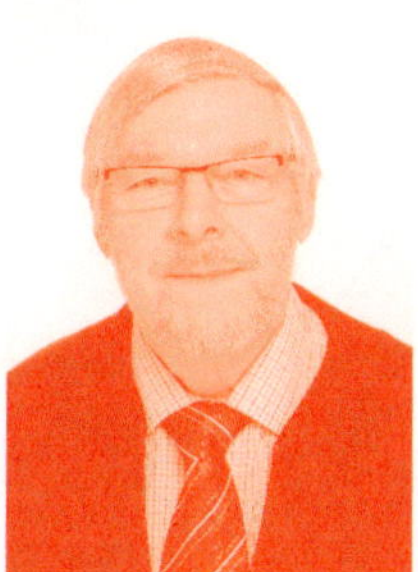
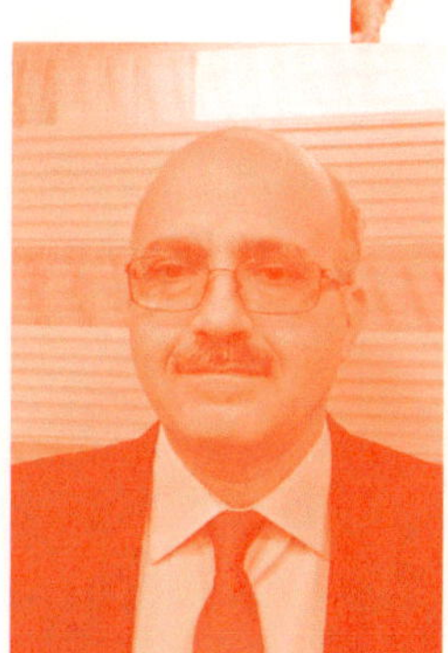
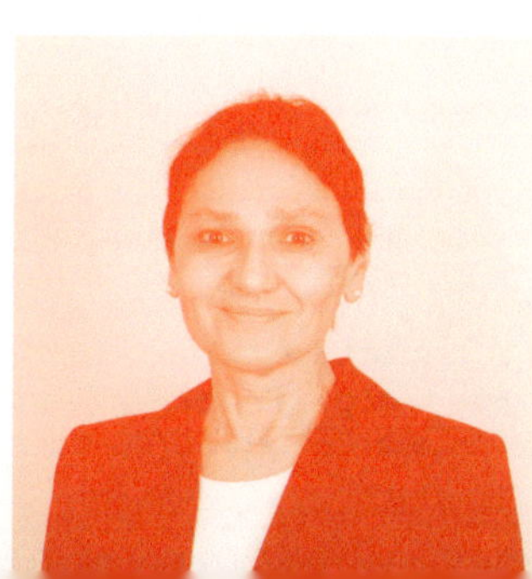
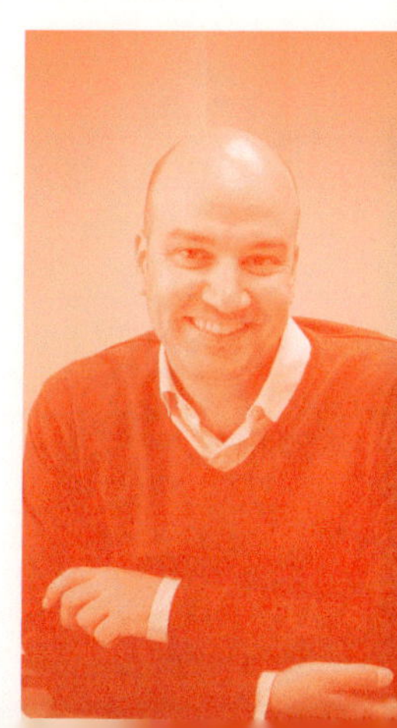

Neurofibromatosis - Current Trends and Future Directions
http://dx.doi.org/10.5772/intechopen.80146
Edited by Francesco Signorelli and Raffaella Messina

Contributors
Hind Manaa Alkatan, Sawsan S. Bakry, Mohammad Abdullah Alabduljabbar, Beata Durcanova, Line Jacques, Andrew Jack, Zachary G. Wright, Vinil Shah, Mina Lobbous, Bruce R. Korf, Brian Potter, Leanne Mendoza, Phioanh Leia Nghiemphu, Donna Molaie, Francesco Signorelli, Raffaella Messina

First published in London, United Kingdom, 2020 by IntechOpen
IntechOpen is the global imprint of INTECHOPEN LIMITED, registered in England and Wales, registration number: 11086078, 7th floor, 10 Lower Thames Street, London, EC3R 6AF, United Kingdom
Printed in Croatia

British Library Cataloguing-in-Publication Data
A catalogue record for this book is available from the British Library

Additional hard and PDF copies can be obtained from orders@intechopen.com

Neurofibromatosis - Current Trends and Future Directions
Edited by Francesco Signorelli and Raffaella Messina
p. cm.
Print ISBN 978-1-78985-529-6
Online ISBN 978-1-78985-530-2
eBook (PDF) ISBN 978-1-83880-576-0

For EU product safety concerns:
IN TECH d.o.o., Prolaz Marije Krucifikse Kozulić 3, 51000 Rijeka, Croatia, info@intechopen.com or visit our website at intechopen.com.

Meet the editors

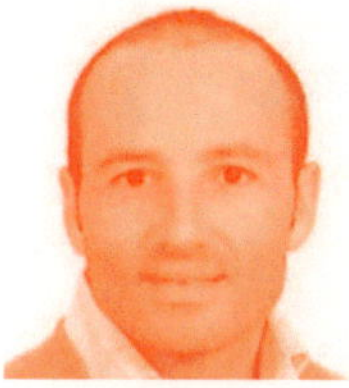

Prof. Francesco Signorelli is an Italian and French board-certified neurosurgeon. He was trained in neurosurgery at the University Hospital of Naples, Italy and was fellow in neurosurgery in London, Southampton, UK, and in Montreal, Canada. He spent 15 years working as a consultant neurosurgeon at the Hospital for Neurology and Neurosurgery in Lyon, France. He is currently professor and head of the Neurosurgical Division of the University Hospital in Bari, Italy. His surgical practice and scientific activity cover the spectrum of neurosurgery, with more than 3000 interventions, more than 60 articles in peer-reviewed journals, and several books. His current major interests are vascular neurosurgery and brain and skull base tumors in adult and pediatric patients.

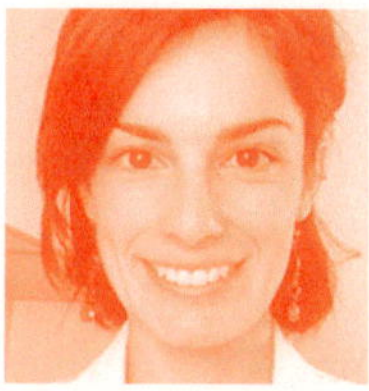

Dr. Raffaella Messina is an Italian board-certified neurosurgeon. She was trained in neurosurgery at the University Hospital in Bari, Italy and was fellow in pediatric neurosurgery in Rome, where she spent five years working as a consultant neurosurgeon at the IRCCS Institute for Treatment and Research – Bambino Gesu Children's Hospital. She is currently consultant neurosurgeon at the University Hospital in Bari, Italy. Her major field of interest is pediatric neurosurgery, in which she has focused her main scientific activity. Dr. Messina had the opportunity to improve her surgical skills and to achieve board certification from the European Society for Pediatric Neurosurgery (ESPN), attending the three-year cycle of ESPN in Germany, Finland and Spain.

Contents

Preface

Neurosurgeons should have a fundamental knowledge of the scientific evidence derived from a multidisciplinary approach regarding genetic conditions such as Neurofibromatosis. Such knowledge can lead to a high level of expertise and properly guide patient management. This book was conceived as an example of the aforementioned integrated approach. Written by outstanding researchers and clinicians, this volume is designed for graduate students, researchers and practitioners interested in learning how knowledge from research can implement clinical competencies. It is hoped that it will stimulate interest in translating research on Neurofibromatosis into practice.

I wish to thank all the authors for their excellent contributions. Without their enthusiastic participation this book would have not been possible. I also wish to thank to Mr. Gordan Tot, IntechOpen's publishing process manager, whose competence and kind patience in stimulating all participants, including myself and my co-editor Prof. Raffaella Messina, was invaluable in finalizing this book. I am especially grateful to my wife Vanessa and my daughter Alice for their understanding and support, allowing me to spend many extra hours working on this book.

Francesco Signorelli, MD, Msc
Chairman and Professor of Neurosurgery,
University Hospital of Bari,
Italy

Raffaella Messina, MD
Assistant Professor of Neurosurgery,
University Hospital of Bari,
Italy

Section 1

Introductory Section

Chapter 1

Introductory Chapter: Neurofibromatosis - Current Trends and Future Directions

Raffaella Messina and Francesco Signorelli

1. Introduction

Neurofibromatosis (NF) is a rare genetic-hereditary syndrome with autosomal dominant transmission and complete penetrance yet variable clinical expression. It is precisely this genotypically defined but phenotypically variable behavior of the NF which is of particular interest as it is able to influence not only the timeliness of clinical diagnosis but also the prognosis of the disease. Indeed, in most cases clinical diagnosis is early (within the first 3 years after birth), but in particular forms with a low phenotypic expression, especially in the mosaic forms of mild neurofibromatosis type 2 (NF2), it can be later, with clinical manifestation of the syndromic features in early adulthood [1, 2].

The known syndromic features of NF, although still framed in the context of rare diseases, differ in their incidence and clinical manifestations. Neurofibromatosis type 1 (NF1) is the most frequent, with an incidence of 1 individual per 2500/3500 live births, without significant gender differences and at least 50% related to de novo mutations [3]. Neurofibromatosis type 2 has an incidence of new cases/year equal to 1 individual for every 25,000/30,000 live births, correlating in 80% of cases to de novo mutations, and a prevalence of around 1/100,000 which has, over the past 20 years, been increasing hand in hand with the introduction of new and more sophisticated diagnostic methods [2].

It is well documented that NF1 is characterized by the presence of an autosomal dominant mutation of a gene on chromosome 17 in position q11, which codes for a protein known as *neurofibromin*, which acts as a tumor suppressor in the pro-proliferative pathway RAS/MEK-MAPK. The total absence of functional protein therefore cancels the inhibitory activity on the RAS proto-oncogene with consequent hyperactivation of the transduction mechanism and the pro-proliferative and pro-mitotic cellular response.

Different mutations have been described on the gene which codes for neurofibromin [4]. In recent years, questions have been raised as to whether the presence of one particular type of mutation rather than another might affect the prognosis of the disease. A study published in Lancet in August 2014 [1] highlighted the possible prognostic role of multiple genomic microdeletions in the context of the entire gene, the presence of which seems to be associated with a more severe phenotypic expression, characterized by the appearance of plexiform neurofibromas at an early age, a significant reduction in IQ, multiple craniofacial anomalies, and a higher risk of malignant degeneration of peripheral neurofibromatous lesions.

On the other hand, the mutation associated with NF2 is autosomal dominant of a gene located on chromosome 22 in position q12.2, which codes for a protein known as *merlin* or *schwannomin* which seems to have a role, not yet fully clarified, as a tumor suppressor in the contact inhibition mechanism of the proliferative stimulus. The alterations of schwannomin seem to be phenotypically expressed exclusively in Schwann cells [5] which would justify, from the molecular point of view, the almost total absence of other neoplastic entities in patients with NF2 or NF3.

Neurofibromatosis type 3, better known as Schwannomatosis, can be considered a variant of NF2 characterized, however, by the total absence of vestibular schwannomas and neurofibromas and by the lower presence of tumors of the central nervous system. NF3 is, rather, characterized by the presence of multiple schwannomas along the course of the peripheral nerves [6].

It has therefore been understood over time that while those gene mutations related to the various NF conditions have complete penetrance, there is considerable variability in terms of the phenotypic expression of the disease, not only between the three syndromic forms of NF but also within each type of neurofibromatosis. Hence the interest of this book, which aims to offer the reader a perspective on neurofibromatosis that goes beyond academic descriptions of what is already known with respect to the different clinical manifestations of NF, instead focuses interest on specific clinical disease patterns, related neurocognitive aspects, and therapeutic developments that in recent years have been emerging in the management of the various types of neurofibromatosis, especially in the direction of new targeted molecular therapies.

As is well documented, the diagnostic criteria for NF1 have, since 1987, been defined by the National Institutes of Health [7], which includes a variable combination of the following manifestations: *abnormal pigmentation of epithelial and mucous membranes* (cafè-au-lait macules, axillary and inguinal freckling, Lisch nodules of the iris); *multiple peripheral neurofibromas*; *bone abnormalities and deformities* (osteopenia, scoliosis, sphenoid wing dysplasia, congenital tibial dysplasia); *cardiovascular anomalies and malformations* (congenital heart disease, vasculopathy, and hypertension); and *neurocognitive deficits*.

Even more variable are the clinical manifestations associated with NF2, whose most commonly used diagnostic criteria are the "Manchester diagnostic criteria" [8]. Such criteria include *multiple central nervous system tumors* (intracranial meningiomas, 43–58%); intramedullary spinal cord tumors (ependymomas in more than 75%); *benign tumors of the cranial nerves* (vestibular schwannoma, 90–95%) that may or may not be bilateral; *peripheral nerve schwannomas*; *ophthalmological changes*; *dermal-epidermal skin tumors of varying natures*; and moreover, a familiar history of NF2.

Following clinical examination and ultrasound diagnostics for skin and subcutaneous lesions, the gold standard in the diagnosis of neurofibromatosis is magnetic resonance imaging with gadolinium of the brain and spinal cord. It has been observed that in patients with NF1, it is not uncommon to locate focal hypointense lesion areas in T1-weighted and slightly hyperintense lesions in T2-weighted sequences, the so-called unidentified bright objects (UBOs), the actual nature of which is still discussed in the literature, although their presence can correlate with cognitive dysfunction [9]. A previous study by Griffiths et al. speculated that they could correspond to areas of subclinical glial proliferation, having hypothesized an association between their early diagnosis in resonance and the relative risk (around 80%) of subsequent development of central tumors of the glial series at between 5 and 10 years of age [10].

Malignant forms of neurofibromas and, more rarely, peripheral schwannomas degenerated into sarcomas are termed as "malignant peripheral nerve sheath tumors" (MPNSTs) and are more frequently associated with the malignant evolution of plexiform neurofibromas more commonly in the third decade of life and with poor prognosis [11, 12].

The treatment of the syndrome is mainly surgical with the removal of both central and peripheral lesions causing functional or evolving damage during follow-up diagnostics. The support that intraoperative neurophysiological monitoring can provide to the surgical resection technique is of fundamental importance, not only for saving the nerve but also in preventing the onset of neuropathic pain. Much more invasive is the surgical resection of MPNSTs, which can sometimes involve amputation or disarticulation to ensure surgical radicalism, followed by adjuvant radiotherapy.

Ultimately, while surgery is still considered the first approach to neurofibromatosis, interest in medical therapeutics for this syndrome has grown considerably in recent years, and numerous clinical trials are still ongoing, as will be explained in detail in the chapters of the book.

Author details

Raffaella Messina and Francesco Signorelli*
Division of Neurosurgery, Department of Basic Medical Sciences, Neurosciences and Sense Organs, University "Aldo Moro" of Bari, Italy

*Address all correspondence to: signorelli2007@gmail.com

References

[1] Hirbe AC, Gutmann DH. Neurofibromatosis type 1: A multidisciplinary approach to care. Lancet Neurology. Aug 2014;**13**(8):834-843. DOI: 10.1016/S1474-4422(14)70063-8

[2] Asthagiri AR, Parry DM, Butman JA, Kim HJ, Tsilou ET, Zhuang Z, et al. Neurofibromatosis type 2. Lancet. 2009;**373**(9679):1974-1986. DOI: 10.1016/S0140-6736(09)60259-2

[3] Anderson JL, Gutmann DH. Neurofibromatosis type 1. Handbook of Clinical Neurology. 2015;**132**:75-86. DOI: 10.1016/B978-0-444-62702-5.00004-4

[4] Yap YS, McPherson JR, Ong CK, Rozen SG, The BT, Lee ASG, et al. The NF1 gene revisited—From bench to bedside. Oncotarget. 2014;**5**(15):5873-5892

[5] Denisenko N, Cifuentes-Diaz C, Irinopoulou T, Carnaud M, Benoit E, Niwa-Kawakita M, et al. Tumor suppressor Schwannomin/Merlin is critical for the organization of Schwann cell contacts in peripheral nerves. The Journal of Neuroscience. 2008;**28**(42):10472-10481

[6] Plotkin SR, Blakeley JO, Evans DG, Hanemann CO, Hulsebos TJM, Hunter-Schaedle K, et al. Update from the 2011 International Schwannomatosis Workshop: From genetics to diagnostic criteria. American Journal of Medical Genetics: Part A. 2013;**0**(3):405-416. DOI: 10.1002/ajmg.a.35760

[7] National Institutes of Health Consensus Development Conference Statement: Neurofibromatosis—Bethesda, MD, USA, July 13-15, 1987. Neurofibromatosis. 1988;**1**:172-178

[8] Evans DG, Baser ME, O'Reilly B, Rowe J, Gleeson M, Saeed S, et al. Management of the patient and family with neurofibromatosis 2: A consensus conference statement. British Journal of Neurosurgery. 2005;**19**(1):5-12

[9] Feldmann R, Schuierer G, Wessel A, Neveling N, Weglage J. Development of MRI T2 hyperintensities and cognitive functioning in patients with neurofibromatosis type 1. Acta Paediatrica. 2010;**99**(11):1657-1660

[10] Griffiths PD, Blaser S, Mukonoweshuro W, Armstrong D, Milo-Mason G, Cheung S. Neurofibromatosis bright objects in children with neurofibromatosis type 1: A proliferative potential? Pediatrics. 1999;**104**:e49

[11] Ferner RE, Gutmann DH. International consensus statement on malignant peripheral nerve sheath tumors in neurofibromatosis. Cancer Research. 2002;**62**(5):1573-1577

[12] Evans DG, Baser ME, McGaughran J, Sharif S, Howard E, Moran A. Malignant peripheral nerve sheath tumours in neurofibromatosis 1. Journal of Medical Genetics. 2002;**39**(5):311-314

Section 2

Peripheral Nerve Tumors in Neurofibromatosis 1, Neurofibromatosis 2, and Schwannomatosis

Chapter 2

Peripheral Nerve Tumors in Neurofibromatosis 1, Neurofibromatosis 2, and Schwannomatosis

Andrew S. Jack, Beata Durcanova, Zachary G. Wright, Vinil Shah and Line Jacques

Abstract

Neurofibromatosis was first described in the nineteenth century. At the time, Friederich Daniel Von Recklinghausen detailed two cases of multiple neurofibromas. Although reports of similar cases had been published before his, Von Recklinghausen is credited with the initial description in 1882, postulating that the tumors originated from nerve sheath and plexal connective tissue. Similarly, in 1822 John Henry Wishart described what is believed to be neurofibromatosis type 2; however, it was Harvey Cushing's description of a case of bilateral vestibular schwannomas in 1916 that highlighted and increased awareness of the disease (albeit the original presentation was thought to be in the context of neurofibromatosis type 1). Since their original description, understanding of these neurocutaneous diseases has greatly expanded. Knowledge of the genotypic mutations and molecular mechanisms underlying the disease pathophysiology has resulted in natural history enlightenment and optimal treatment refinement. However, many aspects of neurofibromatosis have yet to be explained and remain active areas of investigation. In this chapter, clinical, radiological, and surgical considerations for peripheral nerve tumor management in the context of neurocutaneous disorders are reviewed. More specifically, clinical presentations, pathological and imaging findings, as well as management for neurofibromatosis type 1, type 2, and schwannomatosis are comprehensively discussed.

Keywords: nerve sheath tumor, tumor, surgery, neurofibromatosis, schwannomatosis

1. Introduction

Neurocutaneous disorders are a group of diseases characterized by systemic structural abnormalities of tissues derived from the embryonic ectoderm. Among other manifestations, this results in the growth of peripheral nerve sheath tumors (PNSTs). More specifically, of the many diseases that fall under this category, neurofibromatosis type 1 (NF1), neurofibromatosis type 2 (NF2), and schwannomatosis (SWNTS) are the three that predominate when considering those associated with PNSTs. Furthermore, each of these three diseases has a specific gene that upon mutation results in different, albeit overlapping, clinical manifestations [1, 2].

Many different mutations have been linked to these diseases, which may then be inherited (familial forms) or occur sporadically. However, it is the specific genotypic mutation pattern of a patient that will then dictate and drive the molecular pathogenesis leading to their phenotypic disease expression [3, 4]. Because of this, each of the three diseases is generally associated with a particular type of peripheral nerve pathology, including benign PNST (BPNST, whether neurofibroma or schwannoma and the subcategories of each) and/or malignant PNST (MPNST). Moreover, each disease has unique epidemiological characteristics separating one from another. In this chapter, these characteristics, as well as each disease's distinct clinical, radiological, and treatment-related challenges are discussed.

2. Neurofibromatosis type 1

2.1 Background

NF1 is the most common of the three neurocutaneous diseases with a reported incidence of 1:2500–3500 [5, 6]. It is characterized by a somatic or germ line mutation on the long arm of chromosome 17 (ch17q11.2) and is inherited in an autosomal dominant (AD) fashion. This genetic locus codes for the protein neurofibromin and is a tumor suppressor gene expressed in multiple tissues. In short, neurofibromin is a GTPase-activating protein that catalyzes the inactivation of Ras protein (acting as a negative regulator in the Ras/MAPK signal transduction pathway) [6–8]. Its genetic alteration (via point mutations, deletions, insertions, microdeletions, and splicing mutations) results in a loss of inhibition of Ras that leads to hyperactivation of downstream effectors MEK, ERK, and/or mTOR [8]. The latter then results in Schwann cell proliferation and tumor growth. Although NF1 may be inherited in an AD fashion, approximately half of NF1 cases arise from de novo mutations. With more than 500 mutations identified to date, there are also many different types of mutations that can lead to NF1. Although the disease's penetrance approaches 100%, the expressivity of NF1 can be quite variable and may be dictated by the underlying genetic alterations [9]. For example, large complete gene deletions have been associated with intellectual disability, tumor burden, and their malignant transformation [10, 11]. More specifically, the predominant tumor burden that occurs in NF1 patients consists of neurofibromas. Neurofibromas are BPNSTs made up Schwann cells and/or perineurial cells, fibroblasts, hematopoietic cells, among others. After schwannomas, they are the most common type of PNST in the general population with a reported prevalence of 10–24% [12]. Unlike schwannomas, however, neurofibromas tend to be more widespread and occur in a slightly younger population (typically 20- to 30-year-olds) without a clear sex predilection [12–14]. Furthermore, they may occur sporadically or in the context of NF. Those occurring with NF tend to be numerous and, as will be discussed in the next section, of a different histopathological category with a higher proclivity for malignancy.

2.2 Neurofibroma histopathology and subtypes

Neurofibromas are heterogeneous tumors believed to originate from Schwann cells [6, 15]. Grayish-tan in color, they are typically more fibrous and tenacious than schwannomas without necrosis or hemorrhage [16]. Microscopically, poorly organized spindle cells are seen within a myxoid tumor background of coarse collagen bundles. Although somewhat variable, neurofibromas have low-to-moderate cellularity with minimal mitoses compared to their malignant counterpart described below [7, 16].

Dermal (or cutaneous) neurofibromas are a type of neurofibromas with several subcategories. They are believed to arise from a single nerve and may be further subcategorized into localized or diffuse (90% and 10% of dermal neurofibromas, respectively) [10, 17]. Moreover, 90% of cutaneous neurofibromas occur sporadically, while the other 10% are syndromic [18, 19]. Although both are typically unencapsulated, localized neurofibromas are well circumscribed, whereas diffuse are an en-plaque-like growth and less delimited from surrounding tissue. Dermal neurofibromas do not usually require treatment (unless they are painful, bleeding, or interfere with an individual's day-to-day function) [20], nor do they usually undergo malignant transformation [21].

Intraneural neurofibromas are localized, well-circumscribed BPNSTs arising as a fusiform enlargement of a single nerve. Localized intraneural neurofibromas may be seen as occurring cranially, spinally, peripherally, or from autonomic nerves; nerve is intermixed throughout the tumor [22]. Theses tumors are typically encapsulated and present as painful masses that can cause a sensorimotor neurologic deficit. Furthermore, they have an intermediate potential for malignant transformation [10].

Plexiform neurofibromas are complex lesions involving multiple nerve fascicles growing and coming together to make up an entangled neurofibromatous mass ("bag-of-worms"). These occur almost exclusively in the context of NF1 (many considering them pathognomonic) and grow most rapidly during the first decade of life. The most common locations for this type of neurofibroma are paraspinal and plexal areas; however, they may also be seen peripherally (e.g., from the sciatic or femoral nerve) [23]. Overlying these tumors, cutaneous changes may be seen such as hyperpigmentation and thinning of hair. They are also associated with an increased risk of malignancy (MPNST) [17]. An increase in the size, progressive pain, and neurological deficit have all been found to be clinical indicators of malignant transformation and should prompt immediate diagnostic and/or therapeutic management.

Elephantiasis neurofibromatosa is a rare, massive, soft tissue tumor with an intermediate malignancy potential that is exclusive to NF1 (pathognomonic). It is the least frequent type of neurofibroma and consists of diffuse soft tissue enlargement (often in the extremities) with an underlying plexiform neurofibroma or enlarged nerve within the mass [10].

Atypical neurofibromas are simply neurofibromas (of any histological subtype, although certain types display a higher proclivity for atypical transformation) that display histopathological and molecular features involved in malignant transformation. However, they do not fit into a single grading system and more recently they have been termed "atypical neurofibromatous neoplasms of uncertain biological potential" (ANNUBP). These lesions may be destructive locally but are less likely to metastasize [21]. Even though atypia may be present, it is the loss of neurofibroma architecture, high cellularity, and presence of mitotic activity that are more associated with malignant transformation. ANNUBP has its own specific histological criteria for diagnosis; however, the inclusion of "uncertain" within its name argues the need for more research. For example, some tumors exhibit benign, atypical, and malignant features within the same lesion [17]. Furthermore, these lesions can be positive on fluorodeoxyglucose positron emission tomography (FDG-PET) and include areas of hypercellularity and atypical nuclei without increased mitotic activity or malignant change [24]. However, as in the case of MPNST suspicion, diagnosis of such a lesion should prompt more diagnostic and/or therapeutic intervention.

Finally, hybrid neurofibromas are a histological class displaying characteristics of both schwannomas and neurofibromas. Approximately 60% of patients with these tumors carry a neurocutaneous diagnosis such as NF1, NF2, or SWNTS.

2.3 Malignant peripheral nerve sheath tumors

MPNSTs are aggressive sarcomas with a dismal prognosis arising from the peripheral nervous system (PNS) or peripheral nerve sheath cells. Grossly, they are typically fusiform or globoid in shape with a firm exterior and adherent to adjacent structures. Their center is often necrotic, with pseudocysts and evidence of hemorrhage. Microscopically, invasion into surrounding structures, vascular invasion, nuclear pleomorphism, increased cellularity, necrosis, and mitoses can be seen [9, 15, 16, 21].

They are graded according to the Enneking scheme and exist on a histological spectrum (low-grade, benign-like tumors on one end and high-grade, aggressive tumors with invasive and metastatic potential on the other) [15, 21]. Malignant transformation of BPNSTs in the context of NF1 patients is an area of active investigation. Akin to a two-hit hypothesis, mutation of the second neurofibromin encoding allele (or a second, intricately related gene) may be necessary for this transformation to occur [8, 10, 21, 25]. Approximately half of MPNSTs occur in the context of NF1 (one of the most important prognostic factors), and NF1 patients have approximately a 10% lifetime risk of acquiring this malignancy [26–28]. Of the subtypes, plexiform neurofibromas harbor the highest risk of malignant transformation with more than 80% of MPNSTs arising from them. These tend to occur between second and fifth decades of life (peak in third decade) [8, 11, 21] and typically occur at an earlier age in NF patients (second to third decade vs. third to sixth decade in the general population) [9]. Moreover, they are the most common type of malignancy in NF1 patients, as well as the most common cause of death [8]. In keeping with plexiform tumor characteristics, MPNSTs usually arise from large nerves or trunks (brachial and lumbosacral plexus or the sciatic nerve). They also often occur in a deep-to-fascial location (deep soft tissue and visceral tumors frequently being associated with NF1); however, they may occur more superficially as well [29]. As discussed in subsequent sections, MPNSTs are staged and treated as soft tissue sarcomas [8] with previous studies demonstrating a poor 5-year overall survival (OAS).

2.4 Clinical presentation

Neurofibromas are often an asymptomatic, incidental finding. However, when symptomatic, patients may experience pain, patchy anesthesia or paresthesia, and weakness [7]. The incidence of neurological deficit at presentation is higher for neurofibromas than schwannomas; furthermore, unlike sporadic cases, patients with NF1 can present with signs and symptoms from a multitude of different organ systems. Due to the ubiquitous and intricate nature of the Ras signal transduction pathway, the effects of NF1 can be widespread (segmental neurofibromatosis being an exception) [30, 31]. Diagnosis of NF1 is based on the National Institutes of Health clinical consensus criteria (with optional genetic confirmation), and the diagnosis of a neurofibroma (whether sporadic or syndromic, benign or malignant) is a histopathological one. However, the improvement in diagnostic accuracy of imaging investigations such as magnetic resonance imaging (MRI) and PET has resulted in the necessity of biopsies being an antiquated notion. If required, the benefit of a biopsy should be weighed against risks such as neurological deficit and insufficient/non-diagnostic sampling error [9, 15, 17, 21].

NF1 can present with cutaneous changes (café-au-lait spots and intertriginous freckling being reported in >99% and 85% of patients, respectively) [17], Lisch nodules (ocular hamartoma hyperpigmentations), skeletal abnormalities (long bone dysplasia and scoliosis), central nervous system (CNS) lesions such as optic nerve gliomas (15% of patients typically before 10 years of age), brainstem, and hemispheric gliomas may also occur [6, 32, 33]. Moreover, unlike the other neurocutaneous syndromes, cognitive impairment (60% of patients) is also much more prevalent, as is non-nervous system involvement (leukemia, pheochromocytoma and glomus tumors, gastrointestinal tract tumors, and breast cancer) [6, 17, 32, 34, 35]. Patients with NF1 can also suffer from neurofibromatous neuropathy (a tumor independent, symmetrical sensory-motor neuropathy). This results in sensory predominant symptoms including pain and pruritus [4]. This neuropathy stems from a non-progressive and diffuse neurofibromatous nerve infiltration and hypertrophy. Although only affecting 2% of NF1 patients, it is associated with increased tumor burden and MPNST [4, 21].

2.5 Imaging

MRI is the preferred imaging modality for PNSTs [6, 15]. MR neurography can further determine whether a mass is intrinsic or extrinsic to the peripheral nerve and can aid in presurgical planning. In addition, whole body MRI can be used both for screening patients (quantifying initial tumor burden), as well as for tumor surveillance (to monitor for growth and/or malignant transformation) [36]. Signal intensity of neurofibromas is usually low on T1-weighted imaging and high on T2-weighted imaging (although large tumors can display peripheral, central or heterogeneous hyperintensity on T2 imaging). Enhancement can also be variable ranging from none to homogeneous. The classic pattern of enhancement with solitary neurofibromas is central enhancement surrounded by non-enhancing tissue. Isolated, non-plexiform neurofibromas appear as round or fusiform masses with tapering cranial and caudal ends due to continuity with the nerve. A surrounding rim of intramuscular fat capping the edges of the lesion might give rise to the split-fat sign [23]. A target-sign (hyperintense ring of myxoid material with a hypointense center of collagen and fibrillary tissue) might also be present and is more commonly seen with neurofibromas than schwannomas [15, 23].

MPNSTs may arise from solitary or plexiform neurofibromas. MRI features suggestive of MPNSTs include larger size (≥5 cm), peripheral enhancement, adjacent tissue invasion and peritumoral edema, vascular encasement, and metastases. MPNSTs are often irregularly shaped with heterogeneous enhancement, ill-defined margins, intra-tumoral lobulations, central necrosis and hemorrhage, absence of the target-sign, and an apparent diffusion coefficient (ADC) value of $<1 \times 10^{-3}$ mm^2/s [8, 23, 37].

Functional imaging including PET may be helpful for the determination of malignancy, especially in atypical neurofibromas. A semi-quantitative assessment for the determination of malignancy can be done using a standard uptake value (SUV) cutoff [17]. While F-18-FDG PET activity is invariably present in both BPNSTs and MPSNTs, high SUVs favor the presence of malignancy. A SUV ≥4 is indicative of malignancy and can help direct the ideal site of biopsy [6, 8, 38].

Ultrasound (US) examination has also been shown to be helpful in the workup for neurofibromas. US findings may include hypoechoic lesions that are serpentine, oval-shaped, and well-circumscribed with a fascicular pattern. Plexiform lesions can be multiloculated and nodular, whereas subcutaneous neurofibromas often have heterogeneous echogenicity with multifascicular involvement and a target-sign [35].

2.6 Management and outcome

Management of PNSTs is either surgical or expectant in nature (with the role of radiation and chemotherapy being reserved for select cases). Due to the diverse nature of neurofibromas with respect to subtypes and locations, a concise yet comprehensive description of surgical approaches is difficult. However, like other PNSTs, indications for surgical resection of a neurofibroma may include neurological signs and symptoms referable to the lesion (pain, numbness, paresthesias, and weakness), growth demonstrated on serial imaging, questionable diagnosis or malignancy, and cosmesis.

Solitary, localized, and benign lesions can be completely resected for cure with recurrence being rare (excluding syndromic neurofibromas that may be as high as 15%) [7, 9, 39]. However, surgical resection of diffuse, plexiform, and soft tissue-type neurofibromas should rarely be undertaken and only in select cases with clear surgical goals due to the high associated morbidity [9, 39]. Compared to schwannomas and depending on the specific subtype, neurofibroma resection is often more challenging (greater nerve fascicle integration) and is associated with a higher risk of postoperative nerve injury [40]. To help mitigate this, intraoperative monitoring has been shown to be a useful adjunct to discern functional and non-functional tissue [15]. Postoperative motor deficits after neurofibroma resection have been reported in approximately 6% of cases with the incidence of new postoperative deficit being previously shown to be comparable to that of schwannomas. However, neurofibroma resection involved more extensive nerve dissection with a higher incidence of subtotal resection. Furthermore, in their study, Levi et al. showed that 85% of patients had stable or improved function after resection [15]. In keeping with this, in a separate study, all patients with a preoperative motor deficit remained stable or improved after neurofibroma resection [39].

For suspected or established cases of MPNSTs, systemic staging investigations should be done to help establish management goals. Cases should be referred to a tertiary care center experienced in MPNST patient management with an established multidisciplinary tumor board. In the setting of metastases, a palliative surgical resection with chemotherapy and/or radiotherapy is usually undertaken. In contrast, en-bloc surgical resection (with or without pre- and/or postoperative chemo-/radiotherapy) is the mainstay of treatment for localized tumors without evidence of metastases. Negative tissue margins are the resection goal when feasible and represent an important prognostic factor in the setting of high-grade MPNST [41]. However, in the case of low-grade MPNSTs and atypical neurofibromas, the effect of a negative surgical margin is still unclear and must be weighed against the associated morbidity in achieving this [42]. In general, functional reconstruction of surrounding structures is a secondary consideration and, when possible, should not impede surgical resection [9, 21].

In the setting of large tumors for resection, adjunctive preoperative radiation therapy may be used when en-bloc resection is difficult due to size and surrounding structures. This too, however, must be weighed against the increased difficulty associated with operating in an irradiated field. Furthermore, a survival benefit for its use has not been established [8]. In contrast, postoperative radiotherapy for MPNSTs is often required, especially for high-grade tumors or subtotal tumor resection. Again however, although it may limit local recurrence [21, 43], its effect on OAS is more ambiguous. Proton therapy has also been suggested as a potential adjunct [9]. More recent studies have suggested increased local control rates, though an effect on OAS remains to be seen [39]. More controversial than radiotherapy is the role of chemotherapy for MPNSTs. MPNSTs typically only partially respond in a small subset of patients with no significant OAS benefit. More specifically, ifosfamide and doxorubicin have been previously used in metastatic disease or to reduce tumor size prior to surgery [9, 44]. Regardless of postoperative regimen, long-term, close postoperative clinical and radiological follow-up of patients with MPNSTs is essential due to the high rate of recurrence of these tumors [9, 39].

MPNSTs have a dismal overall prognosis [45]. Incidence of local recurrence can be as high as 65%. Previous studies have reported 5-year disease-free survival rates varying between 30 and 60%, and a 5-year OAS rate of approximately 30% [9, 10, 28, 39]. Poor prognostic factors have been previously shown to include tumor size ≥5 cm, truncal/midline location, subtotal resection (for high-grade tumors especially and its role in low-grade lesions being less certain), high-grade and advanced stage tumors, previous radiation, and NF1-associated tumors [28, 39, 41, 42].

2.7 Case presentation

A 42-year-old man with a history of NF1 presented with right buttock and lower extremity pain, accompanied by paresthesias. MR neurogram revealed a right sciatic nerve PNST (neurofibroma) at the sciatic notch and a left hemi-pelvis PNST arising from the inferior aspect of the left L5 nerve root (**Figure 1**). A posterior, transgluteal approach was used to successfully remove the right-sided sciatic neurofibroma with intraoperative neurophysiological monitoring. Clinical and radiological follow-up were planned for the left-sided lesion after treatment of his symptomatic lesion. The patient's pain and paresthesias resolved postoperatively, and he recovered without complication.

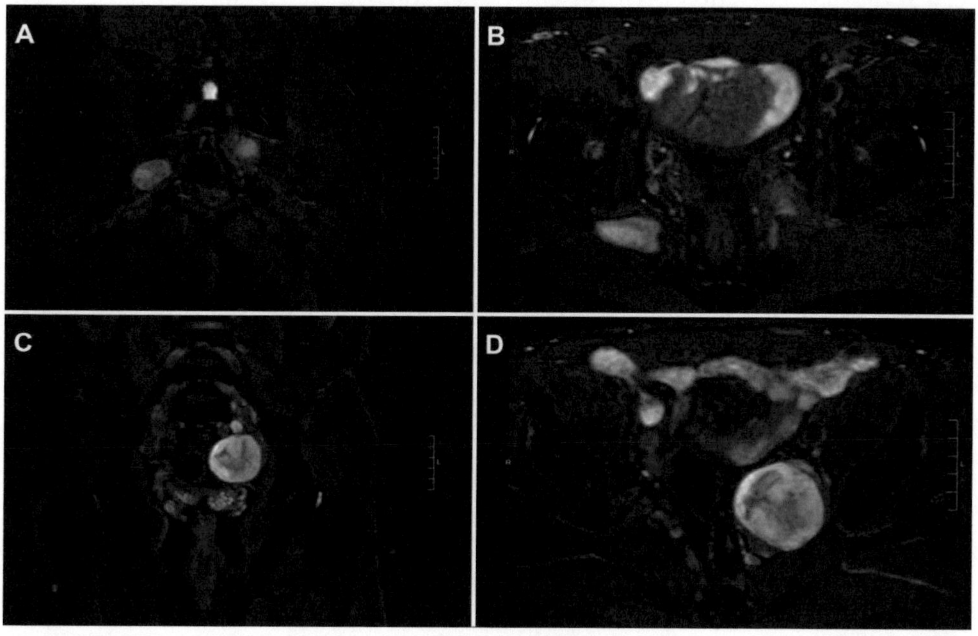

Figure 1.
(A) T2 weighted MRI, coronal section; (B) T2 weighted MRI, axial section; (C) T2 weighted MRI, coronal section; and (D) T2 weighted MRI, axial section. Large round nerve sheath tumor of the sciatic nerve at the sciatic notch (panels A and B), and large left nerve sheath tumor in the left hemi-pelvis, arising from the inferior aspect of the left L5 nerve root (panels C and D).

3. Neurofibromatosis type 2

3.1 Background

In keeping with NF1, NF2 is an AD neurocutaneous disease characterized by a propensity to form craniospinal lesions, most commonly vestibular schwannomas [30, 31]. Its incidence has been reported to range from 1:30,000 to 40,000 individuals. Also in keeping with NF1, NF2 results from a loss of function mutation of a tumor suppressor gene located on chromosome 22q12.2. This gene encodes a protein called merlin (or schwannomin). Merlin is a member of the ezrin, radixin, meosin (ERM) protein family whose function includes anchoring the cytoskeleton to the plasma membrane, interacting with cytosolic elements, and contact-dependent inhibition of proliferation [30, 31, 46, 47]. Through Ras modulation, merlin also acts as a negative regulator of several other transduction pathways [47].

Epidemiologically, NF2 shows no gender, nor racial predilection, and approximately half of NF2 patients acquire a de novo mutation resulting in its expression. Furthermore, 59% of the latter acquire mutation in a somatic mosaic pattern (as opposed to germ line mutation), which portends a better prognosis [47, 48]. Penetrance for the disease approaches 100% in familial patients; however, it may vary in the offspring of mosaic patients [48, 49]. Similar to NF1, specific phenotypic expression and its severity can be dictated by different genotypes; several phenotypes have been described. More specifically, Wishart, Gardner, and congenital types have been described. The Wishart phenotype has the highest incidence and typically displays more rapid disease progression with earlier onset. In contrast, the Gardner subtype is a less severe form of NF2 with onset later into adulthood [50, 51]. A third type, congenital NF2, is associated with dermal plaques in atypical locations, such as the face and hands [51]. The latter phenotype of NF2 tends to be more severe and heterogeneous [46].

3.2 Schwannoma histopathology and subtypes

As their name implies, schwannomas are BPNSTs that develop from Schwann cells and present as well-circumscribed, encapsulated lesions. They are the most common BPNSTs of adulthood and tend to displace rather than infiltrate nerves (fascicles being grossly visible to the exterior of the tumor). Lobular in shape with a rubbery external consistency, these tumors may include cystic cavities, foamy nests, fibrotic and mineralized components, in addition to a hemorrhagic core [4, 52]. Microscopically, two distinct architectures exist: Antoni A and B. Antoni A areas consist of higher cellularity with spindle-like cells and elongated nuclei arranged in palisades (Verocay bodies). Antoni B tumor areas have a lower cellularity with loose reticular fibers in a myxoid background.

Similar to plexiform neurofibromas, plexiform schwannomas are Schwann cell tumors that encompass multiple nerve fascicles coming together into a multi-nodular, loculated growth around the nerves. This subtype will frequently affect the cervical region, brachial plexus, and lumbosacral plexus [48]. They can be grossly distinguished from plexiform neurofibromas, however, by a less diffuse distribution and their typically affecting a single nerve or nerve trunk [35]. Though not pathognomonic for NF2, they occur more frequently in this population.

Dermal or cutaneous schwannomas are masses specific to NF2 patients. They do not occur sporadically or in association with SWNTS and present as a distinct en-plaque-like mass. These lesions originate from neoplastic Schwann cells that expand the parent nerve and infiltrate adjacent structures including the dermis, hair follicles, and sebaceous glands [50].

Nodular are the most common type of schwannoma. They can occur in a myriad of locations and from a plethora of nerves—cranial, spinal, and peripheral [50]. These tumors tend to grow on flexor surfaces more than the extensor surface of extremities, as well as the head, neck, and upper extremities more than the lower. As mentioned, they will typically grow and displace nerve fascicles to the outside of their capsule. The growth rate of these sporadic growing schwannomas can vary substantially; however, it has been reported to be approximately 1–2 mm/year and 3 mm/year in those tumors demonstrating early growth at follow-up (although rates as high as 17 mm/year have been reported) [53].

3.3 Clinical presentation

NF2 patients usually present in the second to third decade of life (mean age 27-year-old with a mean time to diagnosis from symptom onset of 7 years) [47]. Diagnosis of NF2 is dependent on fulfilling the Manchester clinical criteria (although this may not be the most appropriate diagnostic scheme in, for example, congenital and childhood NF2) [46, 48, 54]. NF2 is characterized by the presence of several different CNS tumors, most notably the growth of bilateral vestibular schwannomas (affecting 90–95% of patients and typically presenting with sensorineural hearing loss, tinnitus, and balance difficulties). Other commonly occurring lesions include spinal tumors (60–90% of patients), meningiomas (50% of patients), gliomas, ependymomas, astrocytomas, posterior subcapsular cataracts, retinal hamartomas, and cerebral calcifications [30, 31, 46, 54, 55]. Congenital and childhood NF2 usually present differently than the typical adult onset presentation of vestibular schwannomas (least likely to occur); these patients are more likely to present with a spinal cord tumor, peripheral nerve, or skin lesion [55]. Approximately 70% of NF2 patients will also present with cutaneous and peripheral manifestations of the disease including hyperpigmented plaques, subcutaneous nodules, and neurofibromas (although nodular schwannomas are still more common and tend to occur around peripheral nerves) [46]. Furthermore, although more common in NF1, up to 50% of NF2 patients may also develop café-au-lait spots (typically smaller, less numerous, and paler with more irregular margins) [46, 56].

When they do occur, neurofibromas tend to have a hybrid neurofibroma-schwannoma histopathology [50, 52]. Furthermore, compared to SWNTS patients, NF2 schwannomas are more likely to present in childhood/young adulthood and result in neurologic deficit rather than pain [50]. These tumors have a predilection for sensory nerves with an average rate of growth of approximately 1–2 mm/year (though different lesions within the same individual may grow at different rates) [47, 57]. Finally, non-vestibular cranial nerves (e.g., cranial nerves 5, 7, 9, 10) affect about 50% of NF2 patients [50], and malignant transformation of NF2 (vestibular) schwannomas has not been demonstrated to be higher than the general population in non-irradiated cases [58]. However, aggressive retroperitoneal tumors and spinal SMARCB1-deficient MPNSTs do occur at an increased rate, and malignant transformation has been suggested to be 10 times more likely after radiation treatment [47, 59].

NF2 can also present localized to a particular part of the body or nervous system as seen in mosaic, or segmental forms of the disease. Segmental NF2 presents as a less severe form of the disease [59] and occurs more frequently in sporadic NF2 cases

(20–30% of patients carrying a de novo somatic mosaic mutation) vs. syndromic [30, 31]. This form of NF2 may also clinically overlap with sporadic SWNTS [51].

Akin to NF1, NF2 patients may also experience peripheral neuropathy (66% of NF2 patients) [60]. This typically presents as a mixed sensory-motor axonal peripheral mononeuropathy (not due to mass lesion) in children causing foot drop or wasting of thenar and hypothenar eminences, and severe progressive polyneuropathy in adults [50, 52, 56]. The pathogenesis might involve nerve compression by Schwann cell tumorlets or aberrant non-neoplastic Schwann cells [48, 50].

3.4 Imaging

MRI represents the most precise means of diagnosis [59]. On T1-weighted imaging, NF2-associated schwannomas appear isointense to muscle with a possible split-fat sign. On T2-weighted imaging, target-sign, fascicular-sign, and/or intratumoral cysts may be present resulting in heterogeneous high signal intensity. Enhancement is variable [52]. Internal calcification, hemorrhage, and cyst formation are more commonly seen in schwannomas than neurofibromas. Whole-body MRI can be used to assess tumor burden and distribution of schwannomas for the purposes of diagnosis, surveillance, and optimal treatment timing [46, 52]. MRI adjunct sequences such as diffusion tensor imaging (DTI) may help in distinguishing schwannomas by demonstrating the eccentric location of the lesion relative to nerve fibers. Tractography can also be useful in preoperative planning by demonstrating the nerve fiber displacement pattern around the lesion. The ADC value can be quite variable in NF2 lesions with a minimum ADC range of $0.8–2.7 \times 10^{-3}$ mm^2/s (values <0.9 are concerning for malignancy).

Unlike in NF1 patients, FDG-PET imaging holds little value in the management of NF2 patients and schwannomas.

On US, solitary schwannomas appear as hypoechoic, homogeneous lesions with distinct borders, an oval shape, and the absence of vascularization. Normal fascicular displacement may be seen, as can focal nerve enlargements, hypoechoic cysts and fascicles, and hyperechoic calcifications [35, 60].

3.5 Management and outcome

In a similar fashion to neurofibromas, schwannomas (whether sporadic or syndromic) are typically slow growing and may not lead to neurological dysfunction for many years [57]. Surgical resection of a schwannoma may be indicated in cases of neurological deficit referable to the lesion (pain, numbness, paresthesias, and weakness), growth demonstrated on serial imaging, questionable diagnosis or malignancy, and cosmesis. Surgical treatment in the way of gross total resection is often curative and successful at alleviating presenting symptoms. Rarely does it lead to neurologic deficit, need for parent nerve resection, or tumor recurrence (depending on the location and size, notably vestibular schwannomas) [15, 51]. However, not all lesions are suitable for complete surgical resection (again depending on location, accessibility, and neural involvement, among others) in which case the goal should be maximal safe resection and functional preservation [61]. Schwannomas in the context of NF2 are more likely to result in subtotal resection than sporadic lesions (former tends to include more nerve fascicles and be more adherent to adjacent structures) [50].

Moreover, dermal tumors are not usually resected, unless they are disfiguring or are functionally burdensome.

Careful consideration should be given to the use of radiotherapy in NF2 patients due to the risk of inducing or accelerating the progression of tumors, especially in pediatric patients [57]. However, stereotactic radiosurgery has been successfully used in treating vestibular schwannomas of NF2 patients and resulted in a higher rate of facial nerve preservation [62]. Currently, little guidance in the literature exists for the use of chemotherapy or radiation in the treatment of NF2-associated PNSTs.

In the context of NF2, age of onset is one of the most important determinants of disease severity [46]. The clinical course of the disease is highly variable, but NF2 patients suffer from a shortened life-expectancy by about 10 years [61]. The twenty-year OAS rate has been reported to be as low as 38% [51]. Tumor burden, perioperative complications, and malignancy have been cited as the most common causes of mortality in this group of patients [47, 50, 51].

3.6 Case presentation

A 45-year-old woman with NF2 presented with a palpable mass in her popliteal fossa and pain in the area radiating down her calf into the sole of her foot. MR neurogram showed a PNST arising from the left tibial nerve, ADC values consistent with a benign tumor, and tractography showing splaying of nerve fascicles eccentric to the tumor (as shown in **Figure 2**). Operative resection of the tumor was completed with neurophysiological monitoring being used to identify silent tumor areas and viable nerve fascicles.

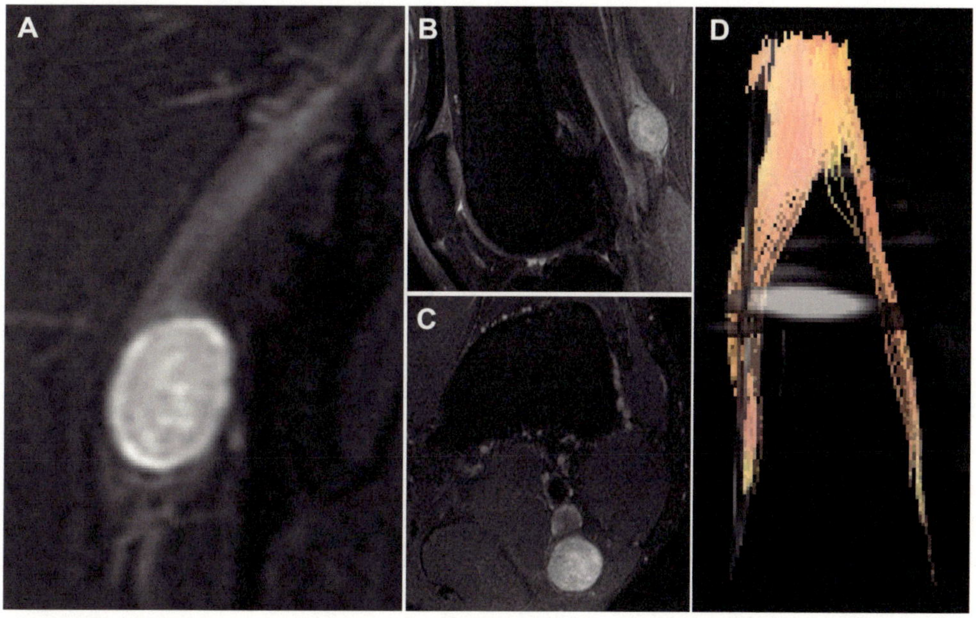

Figure 2.
(A) and (B) T2 weighted MRI, sagittal view. (C) T2 weighted MRI, axial view. (D) Diffusion tensor imaging with tractography reconstruction. Large, round, and well-circumscribed peripheral nerve sheath tumor (schwannoma) arising from the left tibial nerve in the popliteal fossa. Tractography demonstrated intact nerve fascicles being splayed eccentrically posterior and medial to the tumor.

4. Schwannomatosis

4.1 Background

Schwannomatosis is another neurocutaneous disease characterized by the development of multiple BPNSTs, namely schwannomas (in the absence of NF1/2 history). The disease typically has a later onset (second to fourth decade), and some reports suggest a female preponderance [63, 64]. The reported incidence for SWNTS is quite variable; however, many approximate it to be 1:40,000–1:70,000 with a prevalence of 1:70,000–1:160,000 [57]. In contrast to NF1 and NF2, it almost exclusively affects the PNS [31] and can be inherited in a sporadic or AD fashion due to germ line mutation. However, sporadic SWNTS is significantly more common (under 20% of patients having an affected parent), [64] and familial cases generally present at a slightly younger age [63].

As the most common adult PNST, most schwannomas present in the third to sixth decade of life [3]. Many are found incidentally, and due to their slow growing nature, many are quite sizeable before the onset of symptoms (typically presenting with pain and not neurological deficit). The occurrence of multiple schwannomas in one patient should raise suspicion for SWNTS. These tumors can occur in several different locations, including in the paraspinal and retroperitoneal areas, as well as brachial plexus [65]. SWNTS can also lead to the growth of other tumor types such as meningiomas. This, in addition to the presence of vestibular schwannomas in SWNTS, can result in considerable overlap and misdiagnosis of SWNTS as NF2 (especially as mosaic NF2) [57].

Two gene mutations related to chromosome 22q have been identified as resulting in SWNTS—LZTR1 and SMARCB1. Patients with the LZTR1-associated mutation are more likely be affected by a vestibular schwannoma and acquire the sporadic form of SWNTS. Malignant transformation in patients with SWNTS is rare, but does occur. However, mutations in the SMARCB1, LZTR1, and the CoQ6 genes have been implicated in the pathogenesis of SWNTS both in the familial and sporadic cases. Many, as of yet, unknown mutations may also be implicated considering that SMARCB1 and LZTR1 genes were found in only 10% of sporadic and 60% of familial SWNTS cases [66]. Furthermore, in sporadic cases, 55% of the patients did not have their pathogenic variant found, while this was the case in only 31% of the familial cases [40, 57].

4.2 Schwannomatosis histopathology and subtypes

Schwannomas are well-circumscribed, encapsulated, intraneural lesions that most frequently arise from a single fascicle and tend to grow extrinsic to their parent nerve. This results in surrounding fascicles being splayed to the tumor periphery (is in contrast to neurofibromas) [3, 39]. It is not uncommon for multiple schwannomas to occur along the same nerve [67]. Although the majority of lesions are solitary (96%), plexiform lesions do occur (4%) [68].

Morphologically, SWNTS-associated schwannomas are similar to lesions occurring in NF2 or sporadic cases. Namely, Verocay bodies, Antoni A/B architecture, encapsulation, and hyalinized vessels are present. In addition to the above anatomical description of schwannomas, there are also several different histological categories as well. These include conventional or ancient type (commonly displaying degenerative changes such as calcification, cystic change, necrosis and hemorrhage, though usually still follow an indolent course), cellular type (predominantly made up of Antoni A areas, hypercellular with occasional mitotic figures and nuclear atypia, and although may have a higher recurrence rate, still considered benign), melanotic type (comprised of non-psammomatous and psammomatous types with melanin hyperpigmentation and associated with Carney's syndrome; may be or become malignant), and plexiform type (as previously described). Furthermore, mixed or hybrid neurofibroma-schwannoma histopathologic tumor appearance is more frequent in SWNTS than in the other tumor predisposition disorders [4]. Furthermore, although in the absence of radiation exposure schwannomas are not necessarily more prone to malignant degeneration in the setting of NF2, this may not be the case for SWNTS. In a previous study, MPNSTs were noted to occur in 3/181 cases of SWNTS associated with SMARCB1 mutations [69].

4.3 Clinical presentation

The clinical presentation of SWNTS is more non-specific than that of the other familial tumor syndromes discussed [57]. This is likely due to the fact that compared to NF1/2, SWNTS will present with more subtle findings related to slow tumor growth (as opposed to cutaneous manifestations). The most common presenting complaint is pain (focal or diffuse) without neurological deficit, and the presence of a large mass [3, 57, 63, 70]. One previous study found that approximately 60% of patients will have numbness and 30% will have paresthesias at presentation. However, motor deficits are rare [39]. Weakness and atrophy are typically late findings, [64] though they have been found in 12.8% of tumors in one study [39]. It should also be noted that due to mosaicism, SWNTS can also present as a localized, segmental process, which is the case in about 30% of patients [47, 68].

Compared to NF2 patients, SWNTS demonstrates a higher incidence of peripheral nerve and spinal lesions [57]. Schwannomas will affect peripheral nerves most commonly (95%), followed by spinal nerves (75%) with the lumbar spine most often affected [64]. Moreover, cranial nerves may be affected (trigeminal being the most common), though much less commonly [64]. Patients with SWNTS have a significantly lower incidence of meningiomas, ependymomas, trigeminal, and vestibular schwannomas (unilateral still being in keeping with an SWNTS diagnosis) than do patients diagnosed with NF2 [57]. Meningiomas in association with schwannomas do occur, as do isolated cutaneous neurofibromas; however, patients presenting with schwannomas tend to be older than those presenting with neurofibromas for NF1/2 [30, 31]. Diagnosis of SWNTS (and differentiating SWNTS from NF1/2) is predicated on clinical criteria or combined clinical-molecular criteria recently proposed by Kehrer-Sawatzki et al. [71]. However, biopsy to obtain a definitive diagnosis of schwannoma is no longer recommended given the associated risk of neurological injury and increased risk of postoperative neurological deficit after resection [15].

Similar to NF1 and NF2, SWNTS patients can also present with neuropathy (outside of that explained by obvious tumor compression). Patients may suffer from a tumor-independent, intrinsic nerve deficit presenting as a mononeuropathy or polyneuropathy [4]. After investigations are completed, the majority of SWNTS patients presenting with neuropathic pain do not end up having a causative tumor identified. Furthermore, although neurophysiological investigations are often normal in these patients, high-resolution MR neurography has previously demonstrated intrafascicular microlesions. As such, the notion of not finding a causative tumor may simply be an issue of commonly used investigations not being sensitive enough to detect them (tumorlets as seen in NF1/2 being the culprit). Alternatively, an abnormally and diffusely thickened nerve may be to blame [4, 68]. Whether or not these findings are the cause of the pain, and not merely correlative, is another issue. However, SMARCB1-deficient Schwann cells have also been shown to release factors that stimulate nociceptive DRG neurons [4, 61, 68]. These are only a few of the ongoing research areas of SWNTS, as well as NF1/2, being actively pursued.

4.4 Imaging

Imaging characteristics for lesions in patients with SWNTS are similar to those found in solitary lesions previously described. On T1-weighted MRI, lesions appear homogeneously hypo- to isointense to muscle. Postcontrast T1 imaging typically demonstrates heterogeneous enhancement, while fluid-sensitive sequences demonstrate heterogeneous hyperintensity [68]. High-signal intensity on T2 is also usually seen. The use of whole-body MRI is an efficient way in SWNTS patients to evaluate and screen the overall tumor burden, as well as survey for tumor growth or change. With respect to other hallmark features, a target-sign (20%), split-fat sign (96%), tail-sign (36%), and tumor-nerve eccentricity (33%) may all be seen [68].

Although metabolic imaging is useful for malignancy surveillance in neurofibromas, its utility in schwannomas is limited due to the high FDG-avidity of schwannomas, which can consequently mimic malignancy [68, 70].

4.5 Management and outcome

Management for these tumors is similar in nature to that of schwannomas found in other neurocutaneous syndromes. Surgical indications have been outlined above in the NF1/2 sections. Previous studies have demonstrated good outcomes with surgical resection with very low risk of recurrence in the setting of gross total resection. Tumor resection with functional nerve/nerve fascicle preservation is the surgical goal when possible [39, 63]. Surgical removal is typically associated with little to no injury of the parent nerve, in contrast to neurofibromas in which there is a higher associated risk [3, 39]. Resection is carefully performed with removal of tumor capsule unless it is firmly adherent to the surrounding nerve. In the case of the latter, it is left in place. Gross total resection has been previously reported as being achievable in close to 80% of cases peripherally located (versus plexus) [39]. Recurrence of schwannomas after surgical removal is rare; however, it is greatest in cases of subtotal resection and in patients diagnosed with SWNTS (recurrence rate of 14.3% with an odds ratio of 4.29) [3, 39]. A revised diagnosis of NF2 is also associated with a worse overall prognosis. In comparison, SWNTS patients have a higher OAS than NF2 patients (mean age of 76.9 vs. 66.2 years, respectively) [18, 57, 67]. The most frequent postoperative complication is paresthesia; however, motor (5.2%) and sensory (7.5%) deficits can also occur, in addition to neuropathic pain despite appropriate surgical and nonsurgical management (often unrelated to tumor size) [3, 39, 47, 72].

No medical treatments are currently available for patients with SWNTS [3]. However, as for all PNST patients presenting with significant neuropathic pain, neuromodulatory medication such as amitriptyline, pregabalin, and gabapentin should be considered [4]. The use of radiation therapy for treatment of SWNTS-related lesions has not been rigorously assessed and considered only in cases of malignancy or clinically debilitating/unresectable lesions due to the risk of malignant transformation [47].

4.6 Case presentation

A 42-year-old man with a personal and family history of multiple, recurrent schwannomas presented with a palpable tumor arising from the dorsal aspect of the

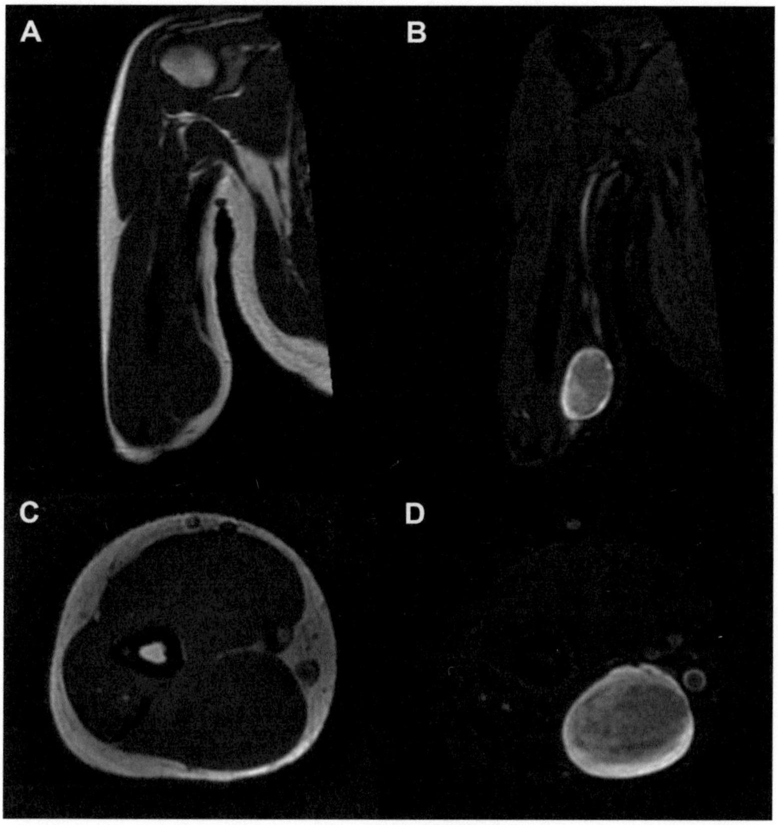

Figure 3.
(A) T1 weighted MRI, coronal section. (B) T2 weighted MRI, coronal section. (C) T1 weighted MRI, axial section. (D) T2 weighted MRI, axial section. Oval, homogeneously enhancing, mass in the dorsal right forearm medial to the triceps arising from the right ulnar nerve.

right ulnar nerve (progressively enlarging since childhood). The mass was located near the right medial epicondyle (as shown on his MRI depicted in **Figure 3**), and associated with painful paresthesias upon palpation in an ulnar distribution. On exam, he had weakness and atrophy of his dorsal and palmar interossei. Operative resection was completed using neurophysiological monitoring to identify silent tumor areas for its safe removal along with the fascicle of origin while preserving the parent ulnar nerve. At last follow-up, the patient's sensory symptoms had resolved, and he had regained some strength; however, his atrophy persisted.

5. Conclusion

Since the initial description of neurofibromatosis (and subsequently schwannomatosis), our understanding of the molecular pathogenesis underlying these neurocutaneous disorders, their clinical manifestations, and respective natural histories has greatly evolved. Technological advancements in areas such as genomic sequencing and radiological imaging have improved both the diagnostic and therapeutic aspects of these patients' care. Despite these advancements, however, substantial work remains in order to fully comprehend the depth of these diseases. It is only through the continued collaboration of research groups and consortiums that these obscure areas will come to light and translate into improved patient care.

Conflict of interest

The authors have nothing to disclose, nor conflicts of interest related to this article, and the contents of this manuscript have not been previously published.

Funding disclosure

None.

Author details

Andrew S. Jack[1*], Beata Durcanova[2†], Zachary G. Wright[3], Vinil Shah[4] and Line Jacques[1]

1 Department of Neurological Surgery, University of California San Francisco (UCSF), San Francisco, CA, United States

2 School of Medicine, University of California San Francisco, San Francisco, CA, United States

3 Valley Children's Hospital, Madera, CA, United States

4 Department of Radiology and Biomedical Imaging, University of California San Francisco (UCSF), San Francisco, CA, United States

*Address all correspondence to: asjack@ualberta.ca

† This author contributed equally in manuscript preparation.

References

[1] Antonio JR, Goloni-Bertollo EM, Tridico LA. Neurofibromatosis: Chronological history and current issues. Anais Brasileiros de Dermatologia. 2013;**88**(3):329-343

[2] Wishart JH. Case of tumours in the skull, dura mater, and brain. Edinburgh Medical and Surgical Journal. 1822;**18**(72):393-397

[3] Barber CM, Fahrenkopf MP, Adams NS, Naum SC. Multiple peripheral schwannomas. Eplasty. 2018;**18**:ic7

[4] Schulz A, Grafe P, Hagel C, et al. Neuropathies in the setting of neurofibromatosis tumor syndromes: Complexities and opportunities. Experimental Neurology. 2018;**299** (Pt B):334-344

[5] Anderson JL, Gutmann DH. Neurofibromatosis type 1. Handbook of Clinical Neurology. 2015;**132**:75-86

[6] Cimino PJ, Gutmann DH. Neurofibromatosis type 1. Handbook of Clinical Neurology. 2018;**148**:799-811

[7] Messersmith L, Krauland K. Neurofibroma. Treasure Island (FL): StatPearls; 2020

[8] Staedtke V, Bai RY, Blakeley JO. Cancer of the peripheral nerve in neurofibromatosis type 1. Neurotherapeutics. 2017;**14**(2):298-306

[9] Garozzo D. Peripheral nerve tumors in neurofibromatosis 1: An overview on management and indications for surgical treatment in our experience. Neurology India. 2019;**67**(Supplement):S38-S44

[10] Longo JF, Weber SM, Turner-Ivey BP, Carroll SL. Recent advances in the diagnosis and pathogenesis of neurofibromatosis type 1 (NF1)-associated peripheral nervous system neoplasms. Advances in Anatomic Pathology. 2018;**25**(5):353-368

[11] Razek A. MR imaging of neoplastic and non-neoplastic lesions of the brain and spine in neurofibromatosis type I. Neurological Sciences. 2018;**39**(5):821-827

[12] Kehoe NJ, Reid RP, Semple JC. Solitary benign peripheral-nerve tumours. Review of 32 years' experience. Journal of Bone and Joint Surgery. British Volume (London). 1995;**77**(3):497-500

[13] Chick G, Hollevoet N, Victor J, Bianchi S. The role of imaging in isolated benign peripheral nerve tumors: A practical review for surgeons. Hand Surgery and Rehabilitation. 2016;**35**(5):320-329

[14] Kim DH, Murovic JA, Tiel RL, Kline DG. Operative outcomes of 546 Louisiana State University Health Sciences Center peripheral nerve tumors. Neurosurgery Clinics of North America. 2004;**15**(2):177-192

[15] Levi AD, Ross AL, Cuartas E, Qadir R, Temple HT. The surgical management of symptomatic peripheral nerve sheath tumors. Neurosurgery. 2010;**66**(4):833-840

[16] Woodruff JM. Pathology of tumors of the peripheral nerve sheath in type 1 neurofibromatosis. American Journal of Medical Genetics. 1999;**89**(1):23-30

[17] Ferner RE, Gutmann DH. Neurofibromatosis type 1 (NF1): Diagnosis and management. Handbook of Clinical Neurology. 2013;**115**:939-955

[18] Bakan S, Kayadibi Y, Ersen E, Vatankulu B, Ustundag N, Hasiloglu ZI. Primary psammomatous melanotic schwannoma of the spine.

The Annals of Thoracic Surgery. 2015;**99**(6):e141-e143

[19] Hirose T, Ishizawa K, Sakaki M, Fujii Y. Retroperitoneal schwannoma is characterized by a high incidence of cellular type and GFAP-immunoreactivity. Pathology International. 2012;**62**(7):456-462

[20] Lott IT, Richardson EP Jr. Neuropathological findings and the biology of neurofibromatosis. Advances in Neurology. 1981;**29**:23-32

[21] Ferner RE, Gutmann DH. International consensus statement on malignant peripheral nerve sheath tumors in neurofibromatosis. Cancer Research. 2002;**62**(5):1573-1577

[22] Brooks DG. The neurofibromatoses: Hereditary predisposition to multiple peripheral nerve tumors. Neurosurgery Clinics of North America. 2004;**15**(2):145-155

[23] McCarville MB. What MRI can tell us about neurogenic tumors and rhabdomyosarcoma. Pediatric Radiology. 2016;**46**(6):881-890

[24] Lin BT, Weiss LM, Medeiros LJ. Neurofibroma and cellular neurofibroma with atypia: A report of 14 tumors. The American Journal of Surgical Pathology. 1997;**21**(12):1443-1449

[25] Korfhage J, Lombard DB. Malignant peripheral nerve sheath tumors: From epigenome to bedside. Molecular Cancer Research. 2019;**17**(7):1417-1428

[26] Miettinen MM, Antonescu CR, Fletcher CDM, et al. Histopathologic evaluation of atypical neurofibromatous tumors and their transformation into malignant peripheral nerve sheath tumor in patients with neurofibromatosis 1-a consensus overview. Human Pathology. 2017;**67**:1-10

[27] Tora MS, Xenos D, Texakalidis P, Boulis NM. Treatment of neurofibromatosis 1-associated malignant peripheral nerve sheath tumors: A systematic review. Neurosurgical Review. 2019 Jun 17. DOI: 10.1007/s10143-019-01135-y [Epub ahead of print]

[28] Vasconcelos RAT, Coscarelli PG, Alvarenga RP, Acioly MA. Malignant peripheral nerve sheath tumor with and without neurofibromatosis type 1. Arquivos de Neuro-Psiquiatria. 2017;**75**(6):366-371

[29] Luzar B, Falconieri G. Cutaneous malignant peripheral nerve sheath tumor. Surgical Pathology Clinics. 2017;**10**(2):337-343

[30] Rodriguez FJ, Folpe AL, Giannini C, Perry A. Pathology of peripheral nerve sheath tumors: Diagnostic overview and update on selected diagnostic problems. Acta Neuropathologica. 2012;**123**(3):295-319

[31] Rodriguez FJ, Stratakis CA, Evans DG. Genetic predisposition to peripheral nerve neoplasia: Diagnostic criteria and pathogenesis of neurofibromatoses, carney complex, and related syndromes. Acta Neuropathologica. 2012;**123**(3):349-367

[32] Gutmann DH, Ferner RE, Listernick RH, Korf BR, Wolters PL, Johnson KJ. Neurofibromatosis type 1. Nature Reviews. Disease Primers. 2017;**3**:17004

[33] Hirbe AC, Gutmann DH. Neurofibromatosis type 1: A multidisciplinary approach to care. Lancet Neurology. 2014;**13**(8):834-843

[34] Al-Adnani M. Soft tissue perineurioma in a child with neurofibromatosis type 1: A case report and review of the literature. Pediatric and Developmental Pathology. 2017;**20**(5):444-448

[35] Winter N, Rattay TW, Axer H, et al. Ultrasound assessment of peripheral nerve pathology in neurofibromatosis type 1 and 2. Clinical Neurophysiology. 2017;**128**(5):702-706

[36] Salamon J, Mautner VF, Adam G, Derlin T. Multimodal imaging in neurofibromatosis type 1-associated nerve sheath tumors. Rofo. 2015;**187**(12):1084-1092

[37] Matsumine A, Kusuzaki K, Nakamura T, et al. Differentiation between neurofibromas and malignant peripheral nerve sheath tumors in neurofibromatosis 1 evaluated by MRI. Journal of Cancer Research and Clinical Oncology. 2009;**135**(7):891-900

[38] Tovmassian D, Abdul Razak M, London K. The role of [(18)F]FDG-PET/CT in predicting malignant transformation of plexiform neurofibromas in neurofibromatosis-1. International Journal of Surgical Oncology. 2016;**2016**:6162182

[39] Guha D, Davidson B, Nadi M, et al. Management of peripheral nerve sheath tumors: 17 years of experience at Toronto Western Hospital. Journal of Neurosurgery. 2018;**128**(4):1226-1234

[40] Chick G, Victor J, Poujade T, Hollevoet N. Sporadic schwannomatosis: A systematic review following the 2005 consensus statement. Journal of Neurological Surgery Part A: Central European Neurosurgery. 2018;**79**(5):408-415

[41] Yamanaka R, Hayano A. Radiation-induced malignant peripheral nerve sheath tumors: A systematic review. World Neurosurgery. 2017;**105**:961-970 e8

[42] Bernthal NM, Putnam A, Jones KB, Viskochil D, Randall RL. The effect of surgical margins on outcomes for low grade MPNSTs and atypical neurofibroma. Journal of Surgical Oncology. 2014;**110**(7):813-816

[43] Keole S, Ashman JB, Daniels TB. Proton therapy for sarcomas. Cancer Journal. 2014;**20**(6):409-414

[44] Higham CS, Steinberg SM, Dombi E, et al. SARC006: Phase II trial of chemotherapy in sporadic and neurofibromatosis type 1 associated chemotherapy-naive malignant peripheral nerve sheath tumors. Sarcoma. 2017; **2017**:8685638

[45] Cherqui A, Kim DH, Kim SH, Park HK, Kline DG. Surgical approaches to paraspinal nerve sheath tumors. Neurosurgical Focus. 2007;**22**(6):E9

[46] Ardern-Holmes S, Fisher G, North K. Neurofibromatosis type 2. Journal of Child Neurology. 2017;**32**(1):9-22

[47] Blakeley JO, Plotkin SR. Therapeutic advances for the tumors associated with neurofibromatosis type 1, type 2, and schwannomatosis. Neuro-Oncology. 2016;**18**(5):624-638

[48] Kresak JL, Walsh M. Neurofibromatosis: A review of NF1, NF2, and schwannomatosis. Journal of Pediatric Genetics. 2016;**5**(2):98-104

[49] Asthagiri AR, Parry DM, Butman JA, et al. Neurofibromatosis type 2. Lancet. 2009;**373**(9679):1974-1986

[50] Coy S, Rashid R, Stemmer-Rachamimov A, Santagata S. An update on the CNS manifestations of neurofibromatosis type 2. Acta Neuropathologica. 2020 Apr;**139**(4):625-641

[51] Ruggieri M, Pratico AD, Evans DG. Diagnosis, management, and new

therapeutic options in childhood neurofibromatosis type 2 and related forms. Seminars in Pediatric Neurology. 2015;**22**(4):240-258

[52] Ahlawat S, Blakeley JO, Langmead S, Belzberg AJ, Fayad LM. Current status and recommendations for imaging in neurofibromatosis type 1, neurofibromatosis type 2, and schwannomatosis. Skeletal Radiology. 2020;**49**(2):199-219

[53] Paldor I, Chen AS, Kaye AH. Growth rate of vestibular schwannoma. Journal of Clinical Neuroscience. 2016;**32**:1-8

[54] Tiwari R, Singh AK. Neurofibromatosis Type 2. Treasure Island (FL): StatPearls; 2020

[55] Lin AL, Gutmann DH. Advances in the treatment of neurofibromatosis-associated tumours. Nature Reviews. Clinical Oncology. 2013;**10**(11):616-624

[56] Ruggieri M, Pratico AD, Serra A, et al. Childhood neurofibromatosis type 2 (NF2) and related disorders: From bench to bedside and biologically targeted therapies. Acta Otorhinolaryngologica Italica. 2016;**36**(5):345-367

[57] Evans DG, Bowers NL, Tobi S, et al. Schwannomatosis: A genetic and epidemiological study. Journal of Neurology, Neurosurgery, and Psychiatry. 2018;**89**(11):1215-1219

[58] King AT, Rutherford SA, Hammerbeck-Ward C, et al. Malignant peripheral nerve sheath tumors are not a feature of neurofibromatosis type 2 in the unirradiated patient. Neurosurgery. 2018;**83**(1):38-42

[59] Evans DG. Neurofibromatosis type 2. Handbook of Clinical Neurology. 2015;**132**:87-96

[60] Telleman JA, Stellingwerff MD, Brekelmans GJ, Visser LH. Nerve ultrasound shows subclinical peripheral nerve involvement in neurofibromatosis type 2. Muscle & Nerve. 2018;**57**(2):312-316

[61] Plotkin SR, Wick A. Neurofibromatosis and schwannomatosis. Seminars in Neurology. 2018;**38**(1):73-85

[62] Chung LK, Nguyen TP, Sheppard JP, et al. A systematic review of radiosurgery versus surgery for neurofibromatosis type 2 vestibular schwannomas. World Neurosurgery. 2018;**109**:47-58

[63] Chen SL, Liu C, Liu B, et al. Schwannomatosis: A new member of neurofibromatosis family. Chinese Medical Journal. 2013;**126**(14):2656-2660

[64] Dhamija R, Plotkin S, Asthagiri A, Messiaen L, Babovic-Vuksanovic D. Schwannomatosis. In: Adam MP, Ardinger HH, Pagon RA, et al., editors. GeneReviews(R). Seattle, WA; 1993

[65] Huang JH, Simon SL, Nagpal S, Nelson PT, Zager EL. Management of patients with schwannomatosis: Report of six cases and review of the literature. Surgical Neurology. 2004;**62**(4):353-361 discussion 61

[66] Elsherif MA, Babovic-Vuksanovic D, Spinner RJ. An association of peripheral nerve sheath tumors and lipomas. Acta Neurochirurgica. 2017;**159**(1):185-190

[67] Chick G, Victor J, Hollevoet N. Six cases of sporadic schwannomatosis: Topographic distribution and outcomes of peripheral nerve tumors. Hand Surgery and Rehabilitation. 2017;**36**(5):378-383

[68] Ahlawat S, Baig A, Blakeley JO, Jacobs MA, Fayad LM. Multiparametric whole-body anatomic, functional, and metabolic imaging characteristics of peripheral lesions in patients with

schwannomatosis. Journal of Magnetic Resonance Imaging. 2016;**44**(4):794-803

[69] Evans DG, Huson SM, Birch JM. Malignant peripheral nerve sheath tumours in inherited disease. Clinical Sarcoma Research. 2012;**2**(1):17

[70] Lieber B, Han B, Allen J, et al. Utility of positron emission tomography in schwannomatosis. Journal of Clinical Neuroscience. 2016;**30**:138-140

[71] Kehrer-Sawatzki H, Farschtschi S, Mautner VF, Cooper DN. The molecular pathogenesis of schwannomatosis, a paradigm for the co-involvement of multiple tumour suppressor genes in tumorigenesis. Human Genetics. 2017;**136**(2):129-148

[72] Merker VL, Esparza S, Smith MJ, Stemmer-Rachamimov A, Plotkin SR. Clinical features of schwannomatosis: A retrospective analysis of 87 patients. The Oncologist. 2012;**17**(10):1317-1322

Section 3

Medical Treatment Options for Neurofibromatosis Type-2

Chapter 3

Neurofibromatosis Type 2: Current Trends and Future Directions for Targeted Biologic Therapies

Donna Molaie and Phioanh Leia Nghiemphu

Abstract

Neurofibromatosis type 2 (NF2) is an inherited tumor predisposition syndrome leading to the formation of vestibular schwannomas (VS) and other central nervous system (CNS) tumors. Clinical NF2 follows a genetic alteration to the NF2 gene, which disrupts the function of a cell membrane-related protein, merlin. Though the role of merlin is incompletely understood, it is predominantly thought to achieve tumor suppressive effects by affecting multiple signaling pathways important for contact inhibition, cellular proliferation, and cellular growth. Patients with NF2 have a bimodal age of onset in children and young adults, with the former tending to present with a more severe phenotype involving multiple tumors. Currently available treatments are non-curative. Surgical resection is the mainstay for growing tumors but comes at the cost of significant morbidity, while radiotherapy is generally not advisable due to the risk of secondary malignancy and malignant transformation. Hence, there remains a critical demand for effective anti-neoplastic therapies for NF2-related tumors. There are currently no FDA-approved biologic therapies for the treatment of NF2. Given the complexity and far-reaching effects of Merlin, multiple molecular targets and pathways have been investigated and are currently at various stages of investigation.

Keywords: neurofibromatosis type 2, Merlin, vestibular schwannoma, targeted therapy, Bevacizumab, axitinib, sorafenib, lapatinib, erlotinib, crizotinib, brigatinib, everolimus, vistusertib, AR-42, selumetinib

1. Introduction

NF2 is an autosomal dominant, tumor predisposition syndrome with an incidence of 1:25,000–1:40,000 [1, 2]. The diagnosis is made based on the presence of specific clinical features. Under the NIH criteria, a patient can be diagnosed with NF2 if they have [1] bilateral VS or [2] have a family history significant for NF2 and any one of the following: unilateral VS, other schwannoma, meningioma, glioma, neurofibroma, or juvenile posterior subscapular lens opacity [3]. Notably, the presence of a pathogenically mutated NF2 gene is not necessary to complete the diagnosis.

The NF2 gene is located on the long arm of chromosome 22, and encodes for the cell membrane-related protein, Merlin or Schwannomin. Though the function of Merlin is incompletely understood, it is predominantly thought to achieve tumor suppressive effects by affecting multiple signaling pathways important for contact inhibition, cellular proliferation, and cellular growth [4, 5]. A wide variety of genetic alterations affect the gene predisposing to NF2, including frameshift, nonsense, missense, and less commonly, splice site [6, 7]. Mutations of the NF2 gene are only detected in 70% of affected patients, and the rate of detection is even less for patients without a family history. This discrepancy is explained by mosaicism: about 25–30% of NF2 patients with a de novo mutation of the NF2 gene are mosaics, where only a portion of their cells contain the mutated gene [8].

Patients with NF2 are prone to develop multisystemic clinical features involving the nervous system, eyes, and skin. The most common clinical manifestations include bilateral VS, intracranial and spinal tumors (other schwannomas, meningiomas, and ependymomas), peripheral neuropathy, cataracts, and cutaneous tumors [9, 10]. Less common but prevalent features include epiretinal membranes, retinal hamartomas, skin plaques, and subcutaneous tumors [9, 10].

The age at clinical onset is bimodal: the first peak is in children, with a median age of onset ranging from 8 to 14 years in pediatric patients [11–13], while the second is between the ages of 20 and 22 for adults [9, 10]. Correspondingly, the clinical presentation of patients affected by NF2 is grouped into two main subtypes: the more aggressive Wishart type, more common for childhood-onset, and the less aggressive Gardner type, presenting in adulthood [13]. Adults tend to present with symptoms of tinnitus, hearing loss, and/or imbalance related to VS, while children have a higher likelihood of presenting with symptoms due to spinal cord compression or other CNS-tumors, as well as ophthalmologic involvement [11, 12, 14].

Growth rates for NF2-related tumors vary [15]. Although NF2-related VS are generally slow growing, they are known to cause considerable morbidity and mortality. Left untreated VS leads to decline in auditory function and complete hearing loss over a period of several years [16]. The goal of treatments for NF2 is to reduce the presence of disabling symptoms, and help improve overall survival for patients. Unfortunately, there are no FDA-approved pharmacologic therapies, and currently available treatment options are non-curative. Surgical resection remains the only approved and standard treatment for NF2-related tumors, while radiotherapy is a less desirable option. Targeted biologic therapies may be an emergent treatment option.

Surgical resection is indicated for VS with accelerated growth rate, ≥3 cm in size, and/or symptoms of radiographic evidence due to compression of adjacent structures [17]. However, surgical intervention comes at the risk of hearing loss, facial paralysis, damage of lower cranial nerves, stroke, and CSF leak [17]. In addition, VS can recur following resection: a large retrospective review evaluating 148 NF2 patients with a mean pre-operative tumor size of 3.1 cm and a mean follow-up of 12 years revealed a recurrence rate of 14% [18]. The size of VS also does not correlate with the degree of hearing loss [19, 20], and at times there is profound hearing loss despite a very small size of the VS where surgical resection would unlikely reverse deafness. In contrast to VS, other schwannomas tend to be slower growing and hence surveillance with serial imaging is recommended; surgical resection is reserved for tumors symptomatically affecting the patient [17].

In regards to NF2-related meningiomas, surgical resection is advised when patients become symptomatic or tumors demonstrate increased growth rate [10, 17]. In contrast, the role of surgical resection for spinal ependymomas is not clearly established. Results from a multi-institutional retrospective review suggest that timely resection in the hands of a skilled neurosurgeon may improve a patients' natural clinical history [21].

NF2-related tumors may also be treated with radiotherapy. There is no formal consensus regarding the role of radiotherapy for NF2 patients with growing VS. The use of external beam radiotherapy for progressive VS in NF2 patients is considered controversial due to the increased risk of malignant transformation and secondary malignancy, as compared with patients with sporadic VS [22–24]. Additionally, patients with NF2-related progressive VS treated with radiotherapy have poorer rates of local control and reduced preservation of hearing as compared with non-NF2 patients [17, 25]. In a large retrospective study by Rowe et al., only 40% of 92 NF2 patients with growing VS treated with stereotactic radiosurgery (SRS) retained hearing function at 3 years post treatment; the rest progressed, including 20% of patients who developed complete hearing loss [26]. Overall, radiotherapy for NF2-related VS is not recommended, and is reserved for surgically inaccessible tumors [3]. Moreover, radiotherapy prior to surgical resection has fallen out of favor due to the observation that radiotherapy makes resection of VS more difficult [3]. Data on SRS for NF2-related meningioma is even more scarce. In general, radiation therapy is not advised due to the risk of creating a secondary malignancy, and is reserved for atypical and/or anaplastic meningiomas [17].

2. Biologically targeted therapies

Current treatment options for NF2-related tumors provide only temporary benefits and there are no FDA-approved pharmacologic therapies for NF2. There remains an unmet need for effective anti-neoplastic therapy of NF2-related tumors. Since NF2-related tumors tend to be slow growing, options such as cytotoxic chemotherapies are not appropriate to treat this lifelong condition, thus molecularly targeted therapies represent a better treatment modality and a budding and encouraging prospect.

Merlin is a multifunctional protein that is involved with the regulation of intra- and extracellular molecules and biologic pathways that are important for cellular structure, survival, proliferation, and contact-dependent inhibition. Increased research efforts have enabled the discovery of various molecular pathways and targets relevant to the pathogenesis of NF2-related tumors. These include vascular endothelial growth factor (VEGF), platelet-derived growth factor receptor (PDGFR), and epidermal growth factor receptor (EGFR), phosphoinositide 3-kinase (PI3K)/Akt, histone deacetylase (HDAC), and mammalian inhibitor of rapamycin (mTOR). The mechanisms of these targets and their pathways are briefly discussed here.

NF2-VS have increased expression of VEGF [27, 28], a powerful mediator of tumor angiogenesis [29]. Additionally, VS are highly vascular tumors, making anti-angiogenesis an appealing option that has been evaluated in NF2 patients in clinical studies [30] and is described in further detail in Section 2.1. The precise mechanism of angiogenesis regulation by Merlin is not known, but a downstream pathway implicating the Rac1 GTPase has been described [31]. Merlin is thought to maintain angiogenesis by regulating Rac1 activity. In NF2-deficient Schwann cells, increased Rac1 activity lead to augmented VEGF levels and more tumor burden [31].

Another growth factor relevant to NF2-pathogenesis is PDGFR. PDGFR accumulates on the surface of NF2-deficient Schwann cells [32, 33]. Increased activation of PDGFR leads to downstream phosphorylation of B-catenin, and subsequent destabilization of cell junctions, loss of contact-dependent inhibition, and increased cell cycle activity [32]. Intact Merlin is important for regulating the concentration of cell surface PDGFR through degradation pathways [34]. In preclinical studies, inhibitors of PDGFR reduced proliferation of NF2-deficient Schwann cells via negative regulation of ERK and Akt [35].

The ErbB family of receptor tyrosine kinases has also been increasingly studied in NF2, primarily ErbB1 (EGFR). NF2-deficient cells have increased levels of EGFR [32, 33], leading to increased cellular proliferation and resistance to apoptosis [36]. Merlin can physically associate with and negatively regulate EGFR by controlling its membrane distribution and subsequent trafficking [37–39], thereby blocking various downstream targets including Raf, extracellular signal-regulated kinase (ERK), and Akt [32]. Moreover, pharmacologic inhibitors of EGFR efficiently revert the phenotypic consequences of NF2-deficiency in several types of cultured cells [37–39].

Merlin is also involved in regulating a number of pathways and intracellular targets relevant to cellular proliferation and survival. In NF2 preclinical studies, loss of merlin activity leads to Schwann cell growth via activation of the PI3K/Akt pathway [40, 41]. Normally, Merlin inhibits PI3K activity, preventing downstream phosphorylation and hence activation of Akt, a protein kinase responsible for proteasome-mediated degradation of Merlin [42]. Akt phosphorylation is also regulated by HDAC; pharmacologic inhibitors of HDAC lead to tumor shrinkage and inhibition of cellular growth in preclinical NF2 studies [43].

In addition, gene-expression profiling of sporadic and NF2-associated VS demonstrated overexpression of the PI3K/Akt/mTOR pathway [44]. MTOR complex 1 (mTORC1) is an evolutionarily conserved protein kinase involved with cell survival, metabolism, and protein translation [45]. In contrast, mTOR complex 2 (MTORC2) regulates the actin cytoskeleton and activation of Akt [45, 46]. Merlin is considered a negative regulator of mTOR. Loss of Merlin function leads to constitutive mTOR signaling in NF2-deficient tumors, including schwannomas, meningiomas, and mesotheliomas. Notably, aberrant signaling of mTOR in NF2-tumorigenesis is independent of PI3K/Akt pathways [45]. In preclinical studies, inhibition with mTORC1 reversed the phenotypic consequences of NF2-deficient schwannoma and meningioma cell lines [45, 47].

In the following sections, specific pharmacologic-targeted therapies and relevant clinical studies are discussed further.

2.1 Angiogenesis inhibitors

2.1.1 Bevacizumab

The use of Bevacizumab, a humanized monoclonal antibody targeting VEGF, has resulted in meaningful imaging and hearing response rates for NF2 patients with progressive VS [28, 48, 49]. Plotkin et al. first showed the intravenous administration of Bevacizumab at 5 mg/kg every 2 weeks resulted in tumor reduction in 9 out of 10 patients, with an imaging response in 6 out of 10 patients, and improved or stabilized hearing (as measured by word-recognition scores) in 6 out of 7 eligible patients [28]. Additional studies with larger patient cohorts have demonstrated imaging and hearing response rates of 39–55% and 45–57%, respectively [48, 49], in addition to improved quality of life [49]. The average time to treatment response was 3 months [48, 49]. Hearing remained stable or improved in 86–90% of patients after 1 year [48, 49] and 61% after 3 years [48]; tumor volume remained stable or reduced in 88–90% of patients after 1 year and 54–63% after 3 years [48, 49]. In a large multi-institution prospective study with 51 NF2 patients, predictors of imaging response included older age: 6 patients <18 years with evaluable VS exhibited significantly reduced responses to Bevacizumab and tended to have faster growing tumors refractory to treatment, as compared with their adult counterparts [49]. Similarly, a small retrospective study evaluating the efficacy of Bevacizumab for pediatric NF2 patients with progressive VS also yielded poor results: none of the seven patients met criteria for a radiographic response, and of the four evaluable patients for hearing assessments, one improved while three stabilized [50]. These observations are in line with previous studies revealing that younger patients have a higher likelihood of developing more severe phenotypes with accelerated tumor growth rates [15, 51].

This constellation of clinical results for adult and pediatric NF2 patients lead to phase II clinical studies evaluating the effect of bevacizumab for NF2 patients with growing VS. In the phase II study by the National Cancer Institute, a dose of bevacizumab 7.5 mg/kg every 3 weeks for 12 months was administered, the results of which are pending (NCT01207687). In the study by Plotkin et al., patients were treated with bevacizumab 10 mg/kg every 2 weeks for 24 weeks, followed by 5 mg/kg every 3 weeks [30]. Published preliminary results showed that 22 patients with NF2-related progressive VS experienced tumor shrinkage and improved hearing in 43 and 36% of patients, respectively [30]. In line with past studies [49, 50], the seven NF2 patients ≤21 years had much less benefit as compared with patients >21 years [30]. In fact, only one out of seven demonstrated a hearing response, and no patients had a radiographic response [30]. Reported adverse events were similar to prior studies [48, 49], and included hypertension, proteinuria, delayed wound healing, fatigue and irregular menses [30].

Unfortunately, the presence of these adverse events can lead to interruptions and even discontinuation of Bevacizumab therapy. In addition, long-term therapy with Bevacizumab is also limited by cumulative toxicities: primarily hypertension and proteinuria, but also, premature ovarian insufficiency in menstruating females. Responses are not sustained off treatment and discontinuation of Bevacizumab has been associated with accelerated VS regrowth and decline of hearing function [48]. The optimal duration of therapy with Bevacizumab for NF2-related VS remains unknown.

Bevacizumab has also been administered for treatment of other NF2-related tumors, including meningiomas and ependymomas. In a small retrospective study involving 15 patients with NF2-related meningiomas, a volumetric response rate of 29% was observed, however the median duration of response was limited at only 3.7 months [52]. Hence the effectivity for Bevacizumab in treating NF2-related meningioma remains unclear. In regards to NF2-related ependymoma, a retrospective evaluation demonstrated no significant benefit for patients with solid ependymomas, however, 7 out of 12 patients who had ependymomas with a syrinx or cystic component demonstrated radiographic and clinical improvements in response to treatment with Bevacizumab [53].

2.1.2 Axitinib

Axitinib is an orally available small molecule multikinase inhibitor of VEGF, PDGFR, and c-KIT (a receptor tyrosine kinase), leading to reduction of angiogenesis. Preclinical NF2 models have demonstrated the relevance of these molecular targets in the pathogenesis of NF2-related schwannomas [35, 54]. Specifically, *in vitro* studies on human schwannoma cells from NF2 patients revealed inhibition of PDGFR and c-KIT activation lead to inhibition of schwannoma cell growth and induction of schwannoma cell death [35, 54]. Recently, these results have been translated into an ongoing phase II clinical trial, evaluating the efficacy of axitinib in patients with NF2 and progressive VS (NCT02129647).

2.1.3 Sorafenib

Sorafenib is an orally available small molecular multikinase inhibitor against PDGFR, VEGF, and kinase-Raf1 (C-RAF). The relevance of these markers for VS tumorigenesis has been investigated in preclinical studies: increased PDGFR activity lead to increased cellular proliferation of human schwannoma cells *in vitro* by upregulating ERK 1/2 and Akt [35]. Expectedly, treatment with sorafenib reversed the PDGFR-mediated proliferation of schwannoma cells, and decreased the activity of ERK 1/2 and Akt [35]. These results were translated into a clinical study assessing the intratumoral concentration and activity of sorafenib in cutaneous schwannomas in NF2 patients (ISRCTN49989464), the results of which are pending.

2.1.4 Highlights

- Bevacizumab has efficacy in treating NF2-related VS, as evidenced by tumor reduction or stabilization, and improved hearing assessments or clinical stabilization [17, 28, 30, 49], in addition to improved quality of life [49].

- The exact dose remains to be determined, variable doses of 5 mg/kg every 2 weeks, 5 mg/kg every 3 weeks, and 10 mg/kg every 2 weeks have all demonstrated effectivity [17, 30, 49].

- As compared with their adult counterparts, there is less benefit in the treatment of pediatric NF2-related VS [30, 49].

- Although well tolerated for shorter durations, cumulative toxicities limit the long-term use of Bevacizumab, and responses are not sustained off treatment [48]. Optimal duration of treatment remains unknown.

- Bevacizumab is partially effective in treating NF2-related meningiomas, although these responses are not particularly durable [52].

- No benefit has been demonstrated for the treatment of solid ependymomas, however, ependymomas with a cystic component or syrinx had a modest response rate [53].

- Axitinib and sorafenib have demonstrated anti-schwannoma activity in preclinical studies [35, 54] and have been evaluated in clinical studies (NCT02129647 and ISRCTN49989464, respectively), the results of which are pending.

2.2 Tyrosine kinase inhibitors

2.2.1 Lapatinib

Lapatinib is an orally active small molecule, reversible tyrosine kinase inhibitor of EGFR and human epidermal growth factor receptor 2 (HER2/neu). Preclinical studies showed lapatinib had anti-proliferative effects on human schwannoma cells from NF2 patients *in vitro*, via downregulation of ERBB2, survivin, and other downstream receptor kinases [55]. Subsequently, in a phase 2 clinical trial for adults and children with NF2 and progressive VS, treatment with lapatinib resulted in imaging and hearing responses in 4 out of 17 patients and 4 out of 13 evaluable patients, respectively [56]. However, audiological responses were sustained in only one patient, and persisted for 9 months [56]. Based on these results, the 2018

Congress of Neurological Surgeons suggested there is Level 3 evidence to support lapatinib monotherapy in reducing VS volume and/or improving hearing function in NF2 patients with VS [57].

In addition, the effect of lapatinib on meningioma growth was evaluated in NF2 patients who received lapatinib in the clinical study described above [58]. Eight out of 17 patients had a total of 17 volumetrically measurable meningiomas and received at least 5 cycles of lapatinib [58]. Increased meningioma growth was observed in patients off lapatinib therapy (9 out of 17), as compared with those on treatment (2 out of 17). One patient had significant volume shrinkage which sustained for 23 months on lapatinib [58]. Hence, lapatinib may reduce the growth rate of NF2-related meningiomas and delay time to progression [58].

In regards to toxicity, in general treatment was tolerable and the most common adverse events were minor including most commonly skin rash, and less commonly fatigue, headache, diarrhea, nail changes, and elevations of liver transaminases without impact on liver function [56]. One patient developed a grade 3 toxicity of delayed wound healing postoperatively, and no grade 4 or 5 toxicities were observed [56].

2.2.2 Erlotinib

In contrast to lapatinib's pan-Erb inhibitory activity, Erlotinib is an orally active tyrosine kinase inhibitor that is selective for EGFR. Preclinical studies demonstrated persistent EGFR signaling in NF2-deficient cells contributes to cellular proliferation, and that treatment with a selective EGFR inhibitor stopped cellular proliferation at a high cell density via contact-dependent inhibition [37].

In a retrospective study, 11 patients with NF2-related progressive VS ineligible for surgical resection or radiotherapy were treated with erlotinib on the basis of compassionate use [59]. Unfortunately, no significant imaging or hearing responses were observed, though median time to clinical progression was 9.2 months [59]. Notably, the subset of four evaluable patients reported to experience stable disease on erlotinib all had slow VS growth rates (baseline annual volumetric growth rate ranging from 6 to 14%) prior to erlotinib initiation [59]. In summation, erlotinib is not effective in treating fast growing VS, however it may delay time to progression in patients with slow growing VS. The adverse event profile of erlotinib is similar to that of lapatinib, and primarily included minor toxicities of skin rash, diarrhea, and hair thinning [59]. Two patients developed a rare corneal keratopathy that was related to eyelash curling [59].

2.2.3 Crizotinib

Crizotinib is an orally active, small molecule multi-target tyrosine kinase inhibitor of mesenchymal-epithelial transition (MET), anaplastic lymphoma kinase (ALK), and c-ros oncogene 1 (ROS1). In orthotopic mouse models of NF2, treatment with crizotinib resulted in slower growth of VS as compared with those who did not receive the drug [60]. Kissil et al. found that wildtype focal adhesion kinase (FAK1) was necessary for proliferation of NF2-null Schwann cells and treatment with crizotinib lead to inhibition of FAK1 and significantly reduced proliferation of NF2-null Schwann cells [60]. Conversely, treatment with crizotinib-resistant forms of FAK1 reversed the anti-proliferative benefits seen with wildtype FAK1 [60]. Hence, the primary anti-proliferative activity of crizotinib on NF2-null Schwann cells is mediated through inhibition of FAK1 [60]. FAK has previously been recognized as a target involved with NF2-mediated tumorigenesis [61]. In addition, MET has also been implicated in the pathogenesis of NF2-related VS [62, 63]. Recently, these results have been translated into an upcoming phase II clinical trial evaluating the efficacy of Crizotinib in children and adults with NF2 and progressive VS, set to open for enrollment later this year.

2.2.4 Brigatinib

Brigatinib is an orally available, small molecule tyrosine kinase inhibitor of ALK and EGFR. Based on a cell viability screen, ALK was identified as a promising target for inhibiting growth of NF2-deficient Schwann cells [64]. Subsequently, administration of brigatinib to NF2 mouse models delayed growth of schwannomas and better preserved hearing, as compared with vehicle-treated models [64]. These results have contributed to the development of a phase II clinical study for NF2 patients, which is currently being developed and set to open for enrollment later this year.

2.2.5 Highlights

- Lapatinib has modest effect in reducing VS volume and/or improving hearing function in NF2 patients with VS [56, 57]

- Erlotinib is not effective in shrinking VS or improving hearing function, however, it may delay time to progression in patients with slow growing VS [59].

- Crizotinib and Brigatinib have demonstrated anti-schwannoma activity in preclinical studies and these results have been translated into a phase II clinical studies set to open later this year.

2.3 Mammalian target of Rapamycin (mTOR) inhibitors

2.3.1 Everolimus (RAD001)

Everolimus is an orally available inhibitor of mTOR complex 1 (mTORC1). Merlin is considered a negative regulator of mTORC1, and loss of merlin function leads to increased mTOR signaling and NF2-related tumorigenesis [65]. In preclinical studies, inhibition of mTORC1 with rapamycin lead to VS tumor shrinkage *in vivo* [47] and halted growth of NF2-deficient meningioma cells *in vitro* [45]. These results were subsequently translated into two phase II clinical trials evaluating the efficacy of everolimus in NF2 patients with progressive VS [66, 67]. Both trials included adult and pediatric NF2 patients and subjects were treated with everolimus at 10 mg/day for continuous 28-day cycles. Neither study demonstrated any appreciable tumor shrinkage or hearing improvement after treatment with everolimus [66, 67]. However, in the phase II study by Karajannis et al., three adult patients did experience mild reductions in their target VS (-3.6 to -11.93 cm^3 reduction from baseline); two of these patients discontinued treatment at 3 and 6 months due to personal preference, while the third continued for 12 months with stabilization of their index VS [67]. Goutagny et al. also found that treatment with everolimus resulted in stabilization of tumor volumes, as well as hearing function, in five out of nine evaluable adult patients [66]. Stabilization was parallel to a decrease in the median annual growth rate of VS, from 67% per year before treatment to 0.5% per year during treatment [66]. Overall, time to tumor progression also increased, from 4.2 months before treatments to >12 months with treatment [66].

In the five patients with stabilization of disease on everolimus, discontinuation after 12 months lead to rebound effects on tumor growth rate [66]. All five patients experienced marked growth of VS volumes 2–6 months after discontinuation; one patient had concomitant decline of hearing and balance and elected to undergo surgical resection [66]. In the other four patients, resumption of everolimus leads to a median VS volume reduction of 6.8% at 24 months and increased time to tumor progression [68]. Thereafter, the study was amended to increase duration of therapy with everolimus for another 2 years [68]. At 4-year follow-up, one patient continued to remain stable on everolimus, and the other three patients progressed radiographically after 36, 39, and 45 months of treatment; hearing function was stable for three out of four patients [68]. Hence, reintroduction of everolimus resulted in delayed time to progression from a median of 2.9 months before treatment, to 13.9 months with treatment [68]. In addition, the previously observed rebound effect on VS growth rate following withdrawal of everolimus, did not occur with discontinuation of therapy after VS progression on treatment [68]. Two of the three patients with progression went on to receive bevacizumab, which resulted in tumor shrinkage for one patient and stabilization for the other [68].

Notably, the patients in the study by Goutagny et al. had received less prior medical therapies as compared with Karajannis et al., potentially reflecting a less refractory group of NF2-related VS. No rebound effects were observed by Karajannis et al., however, as seven out of nine patients were previously treated with lapatinib and/or bevacizumab, these therapies may lead to genetic alterations of VS tumorigenesis prior to everolimus therapy [67].

Everolimus monotherapy also resulted in stabilization of meningiomas in NF2 patients. Two patients with asymptomatic frontal meningiomas had increased time to progression of meningioma while on everolimus, from 5.5 and 8.5 months before therapy, to 17.3 months and not reached, respectively, after 26 months of treatment with everolimus [68].

Overall the side effects due to everolimus were tolerable and mostly minor grade 1 or 2 events including mouth ulcers, rash, headache, fatigue, cholesterol elevation, sinusitis, and delayed wound healing [66, 67]. One patient developed a grade 3 toxicity of basocellular carcinoma which did not require additional treatment beyond excision [66] and another had transient azoospermia which resolved after drug discontinuation [67].

2.3.2 Vistusertib (AZD2014)

AZD2014 is an orally available dual inhibitor of mTOR complex 1 and 2 (mTORC1/2). Plotkin et al. found that combined mTORC1/2 inhibition was more effective than single mTORC1 inhibition in reducing proliferation of NF2-deficient meningioma cells in vitro [69]. These results were translated into a phase II clinical study for NF2 patients with growing or symptomatic meningiomas; the trial is active however it is not currently recruiting patients according to cancer.gov (NCT02831257).

2.3.3 Highlights

- Everolimus is effective in stabilizing VS and delaying time to tumor progression in about 50% of patients [66]; these observations are more notable for patients who have not been previously treated with other biologic agents [66, 67].

- Early discontinuation of everolimus in patients' with stable disease may result in a life-threatening rebound effect on VS growth rate [66] which can be rescued by reintroduction of everolimus [68].

- Notably, this rebound effect was not observed in patients who progressed on everolimus [68] or who had been previously treated with lapatinib or bevacizumab [66]. Hence discontinuation of everolimus in setting of ongoing VS stabilization is not recommended [68].
- While the timing of everolimus administration remains unclear, data suggest it is more likely to achieve tumor stabilization prior to other biologic agents [66, 67], and that bevacizumab can be safely administered after progression on everolimus with some stabilization of VS [68].
- Everolimus can also slow the growth of meningiomas in NF2 patients [68].
- Vistusertib is a dual mTORC1/2 inhibitor and may have more anti-meningioma activity than mTORC1 inhibitors [69]; it is currently being evaluated in a phase II clinical study (NCT02831257).

2.4 Histone deacetylase (HDAC) inhibitors

2.4.1 AR-42

AR-42 is an orally active inhibitor of HDAC with multiple downstream molecular targets, including downregulation of phosphorylated-Akt [70], a protein kinase important for cellular apoptosis. Preclinical studies with AR-42 on schwannoma and meningioma cells *in vitro* demonstrated a dose-dependent inhibitory effect on the cellular proliferation and increased cellular apoptosis, by reducing Akt activation [43]. Subsequently these findings were replicated in schwannoma mice xenograft models, which demonstrated the mice that ate AR-42 had 42% smaller tumor volume and less phosphorylated-Akt as compared with those that did not receive drug [43]. Collectively, these studies demonstrate AR-42 has anti-neoplastic activity against schwannoma and meningioma cells via a dose-dependent suppression of phosphorylated-Akt [43]. These results have been translated into a proof of concept phase 0 study assessing expression of phosphorylated-Akt of VS and meningiomas in adults receiving AR-42 prior to surgical resection (NCT02282917).

2.5 Mitogen-activated protein kinase (MEK) inhibitors

2.5.1 Selumetinib (AZD6244)

Selumetinib is an orally available small molecule inhibitor of MEK 1 and 2. The Ras/MEK/extracellular signal-related kinase (ERK) pathway is implicated in NF2 tumorigenesis and is strongly activated in NF2-deficient schwannoma cell lines [71]. In preclinical studies, inhibition of MEK 1 and 2 with selumetinib lead to cessation of cellular proliferation of human schwannoma cells *in vitro* and interruption of PDFGR-mediated ERK activation [72]. These findings lead to phase II clinical study assessing the efficacy of selumetinib for patients with NF2-related tumors, and are actively recruiting according to clinicaltrials.gov (NCT03095248).

3. Conclusions

NF2 is a tumor predisposition syndrome that leads to the formation of VS, meningiomas, ependymomas, and a variety of ophthalmologic and cutaneous features. The management of NF2-related tumors has primarily been with surgery and radiotherapy. However, surgical resection is associated with considerable morbidity, and radiotherapy is increasingly less advised due to the risk of malignant transformation and secondary malignancies. Hence, there remains a critical need for the treatment of patients with NF2-related tumors.

Biologically targeted therapies are an emerging and promising role. Dysfunctioning Merlin underlies NF2-associated tumorigenesis and is a multifunctioning protein intimately involved with molecular targets and pathways important for cellular metabolism, structure, proliferation, survival, and contact-dependent inhibition. Targets that have been validated in preclinical models and translated into clinical trials include VEGF, PDGFR, VEGF, PI3K/Akt, HDAC, mTOR, ALK, and Ras/Raf/MEK/ERK. Ongoing studies for patients with NF2-related tumors include AR-42, selumetinib, and vistusertib, and two other clinical trials are set to open later this year: crizotinib and brigatinib. Currently published results from clinical studies suggest bevacizumab, everolimus, and lapatinib have some effectivity in stabilizing NF2-VS and to a lesser degree, NF2-meningiomas. Bevacizumab, especially, has the ability to preserve function and prevent hearing loss in NF2 patients with progressive VS growth or hearing loss. However, these results are not durable and tumor growth eventually occurs. Given the multifunctioning reaches of Merlin, and the eventual drug-resistance of NF2-related tumors seen with monotherapy, developing a multi-drug regimen may be necessary for reducing the emergence of drug-resistant tumor cells, optimizing cell kill, and improving overall survival.

In summary, major advancements in understanding NF2 biology has enabled the translation of biologically targeted therapies for NF2-related tumors. Secondarily, monotherapy with some agents has resulted in stabilization of disease and clinical improvement. However, these results are not sustained off treatment, are limited by cumulative toxicities, and unfortunately, eventual growth occurs on monotherapy. A multi-drug regimen may be the key to overpowering the multifunctioning reaches of Merlin, and developing more efficacious long-term therapies with improved survival outcomes for patients with NF2.

Conflict of interest

The authors declare no conflict of interest.

Author details

Donna Molaie and Phioanh Leia Nghiemphu*
Department of Neurology, Neuro-Oncology Program, University of California, Los Angeles, USA

*Address all correspondence to: leian@ucla.edu

References

[1] Evans DGR, Huson SM, Donnai D, Neary W, Blair V, Teare D, et al. A genetic study of type 2 neurofibromatosis in the United Kingdom. I. Prevalence, mutation rate, fitness, and confirmation of maternal transmission effect on severity. Journal of Medical Genetics. 1992;**29**(12):841-846

[2] Evans DGR, Moran A, King A, Saeed S, Gurusinghe N, Ramsden R. Incidence of vestibular schwannoma and neurofibromatosis 2 in the North west of England over a 10-year period: Higher incidence than previously thought. Otology & Neurotology. 2005;**26**:93-97

[3] Ruggieri M, Praticò AD, Serra A, Maiolino L, Cocuzza S, Di Mauro P, et al. Childhood neurofibromatosis type 2 (NF2) and related disorders: From bench to bedside and biologically targeted therapies. Acta Oto-Laryngologica. 2016;**36**(5):345-367. Available from: http://www.ncbi.nlm.nih.gov/pubmed/27958595

[4] Cooper J, Giancotti FG. Molecular insights into NF2/Merlin tumor suppressor function. FEBS Letters. 2014;**588**(16):2743-2752 Available from: http://www.ncbi.nlm.nih.gov/pubmed/24726726

[5] Li W, Cooper J, Karajannis MA, Giancotti FG. Merlin: A tumour suppressor with functions at the cell cortex and in the nucleus. EMBO Reports. 2012;**13**(3):204-215. Available from: http://www.ncbi.nlm.nih.gov/pubmed/22482125

[6] Ruttledge MH, Andermann AA, Phelan CM, Claudio JO, Han FY, Chretien N, et al. Type of mutation in the neurofibromatosis type 2 gene (NF2) frequently determines severity of disease. American Journal of Human Genetics. 1996;**59**(2):331-342. Available from: http://www.ncbi.nlm.nih.gov/pubmed/8755919

[7] Plotkin SR. Neurofibromatosis type 2. In: Encyclopedia of Neuroscience. Academic Press; 2009. pp. 419-425. Available from: https://www.sciencedirect.com/science/article/pii/B9780080450469015151

[8] Evans DGR, Ramsden RT, Shenton A, Gokhale C, Bowers NL, Huson SM, et al. Mosaicism in neurofibromatosis type 2: An update of risk based on uni/bilaterality of vestibular schwannoma at presentation and sensitive mutation analysis including multiple ligation-dependent probe amplification. Journal of Medical Genetics. 2007;**44**(7):424-428. Available from: http://www.ncbi.nlm.nih.gov/pubmed/17307835

[9] Evans DGR. Neurofibromatosis type 2 (NF2): A clinical and molecular review. Orphanet Journal of Rare Diseases. 2009;**4**(1):16. Available from: https://ojrd.biomedcentral.com/articles/10.1186/1750-1172-4-16

[10] Asthagiri AR, Parry DM, Butman JA, Kim HJ, Tsilou ET, Zhuang Z, et al. Neurofibromatosis type 2. Lancet. 2009;**373**(9679):1974-1986. Available from: http://www.ncbi.nlm.nih.gov/pubmed/19476995

[11] Ardern-Holmes S, Fisher G, North K. Neurofibromatosis type 2. Journal of Child Neurology. 2017;**32**(1):9-22. Available from: http://journals.sagepub.com/doi/10.1177/0883073816666736

[12] Evans DG, Birch JM, Ramsden RT. Paediatric presentation of type 2 neurofibromatosis. Archives of Disease in Childhood. 1999;**81**(6):496-499. Available from: http://www.ncbi.nlm.nih.gov/pubmed/10569966

[13] Ruggieri M, Iannetti P, Polizzi A, La Mantia I, Spalice A, Giliberto O, et al.

Earliest clinical manifestations and natural history of Neurofibromatosis type 2 (NF2) in childhood: A study of 24 patients. Neuropediatrics. 2005;**36**(1):21-34. Available from: http://www.thieme-connect.de/DOI/DOI?10.1055/s-2005-837581

[14] Nunes F, MacCollin M. Neurofibromatosis 2 in the pediatric population. Journal of Child Neurology. 2003;**18**(10):718-724. Available from: http://journals.sagepub.com/doi/10.1177/08830738030180101301

[15] Peyre M, Goutagny S, Bah A, Bernardeschi D, Larroque B, Sterkers O, et al. Conservative Management of Bilateral Vestibular Schwannomas in Neurofibromatosis type 2 patients. Neurosurgery. 2013;**72**(6):907-914. Available from: https://academic.oup.com/neurosurgery/article-lookup/doi/10.1227/NEU.0b013e31828bae28

[16] Black P, Loeffler J. Cancer of the Nervous System—Google Books. Second. Baltimore, New York, London: Lippincott Williams and Wilkins; 2004. pp. 403-406. Available from: https://books.google.com/books?id=CTGXvRvKO2kC&pg=PA404&lpg=PA404&dq=nf2+vs+fluctuating+growth+rate&source=bl&ots=Zbcs26czuw&sig=ACfU3U1dtBeVHrqY3_uzobKkhVGriMGMRw&hl=en&sa=X&ved=2ahUKEwiugbyin-fjAhVUs54KHabIB78Q6AEwDXoECAkQAQ#v=onepage&q=nf2vsfluct

[17] Blakeley JO, Evans DG, Adler J, Brackmann D, Chen R, Ferner RE, et al. Consensus recommendations for current treatments and accelerating clinical trials for patients with neurofibromatosis type 2. American Journal of Medical Genetics. Part A. 2012;**158A**(1):24-41. Available from: http://www.ncbi.nlm.nih.gov/pubmed/22140088

[18] Moffat DA, Lloyd SKW, Macfarlane R, Mannion R, King A, Rutherford S, et al. Outcome of translabyrinthine surgery for vestibular schwannoma in neurofibromatosis type 2. British Journal of Neurosurgery. 2013;**27**(4):446-453

[19] Arriaga MA, Long S, Nelson R. Clinical correlates of acoustic neuroma volume. The American Journal of Otology. 1993;**14**(5):465-468. Available from: http://www.ncbi.nlm.nih.gov/pubmed/8122709

[20] Nadol JB, Diamond PF, Thornton AR. Correlation of hearing loss and radiologic dimensions of vestibular schwannomas (acoustic neuromas). The American Journal of Otology. 1996;**17**(2):312-316

[21] Kalamarides M, Essayed W, Lejeune JP, Aboukais R, Sterkers O, Bernardeschi D, et al. Spinal ependymomas in NF2: A surgical disease? Journal of Neuro-Oncology. 2018;**136**(3):605-611. Available from: https://doi.org/10.1007/s11060-017-2690-7

[22] Baser ME, Evans DG, Jackler RK, Sujansky E, Rubenstein A. Neurofibromatosis 2, radiosurgery and malignant nervous system tumours. British Journal of Cancer. 2000;**82**(4):998-998. Available from: http://www.ncbi.nlm.nih.gov/pubmed/10732777

[23] Evans DGR, Birch JM, Ramsden RT, Sharif S, Baser ME. Malignant transformation and new primary tumours after therapeutic radiation for benign disease: Substantial risks in certain tumour prone syndromes. Journal of Medical Genetics. 2006;**43**(4):289-294. Available from: http://www.ncbi.nlm.nih.gov/pubmed/16155191

[24] Balasubramaniam A, Shannon P, Hodaie M, Laperriere N, Michaels H, Guha A. Glioblastoma multiforme after stereotactic radiotherapy for acoustic neuroma: Case report and review

of the literature. Neuro-Oncology. 2007;**9**(4):447-453. Available from: http://www.ncbi.nlm.nih.gov/pubmed/17704364

[25] Anderson BM, Khuntia D, Bentzen SM, Geye HM, Hayes LL, Kuo JS, et al. Single institution experience treating 104 vestibular schwannomas with fractionated stereotactic radiation therapy or stereotactic radiosurgery. Journal of Neuro-Oncology. 2014;**116**(1):187-193. Available from: http://link.springer.com/10.1007/s11060-013-1282-4

[26] Rowe J, Radatz M, Kemeny A. Modern Management of Acoustic Neuroma. Progress Neurological Surgery. Vol. 21. Basel, Karger. UK: Jeremy Rowe National Centre for Stereotactic Radiosurgery, Royal Hallamshire Hospital; 2008. Available from: https://www.karger.com/Article/Pdf/156907

[27] Uesaka T, Shono T, Suzuki SO, Nakamizo A, Niiro H, Mizoguchi M, et al. Expression of VEGF and its receptor genes in intracranial schwannomas. Journal of Neuro-Oncology. 2007;**83**(3):259-266. Available from: http://link.springer.com/10.1007/s11060-007-9336-0

[28] Plotkin SR, Stemmer-Rachamimov AO, Barker FG, Halpin C, Padera TP, Tyrrell A, et al. Hearing improvement after Bevacizumab in patients with Neurofibromatosis type 2. The New England Journal of Medicine. 2009;**361**(4):358-367. Available from: http://www.nejm.org/doi/abs/10.1056/NEJMoa0902579

[29] Simons M, Gordon E, Claesson-Welsh L. Mechanisms and regulation of endothelial VEGF receptor signalling. Nature Reviews. Molecular Cell Biology. 2016;**17**(10):611-625. Available from: http://www.nature.com/articles/nrm.2016.87

[30] Plotkin SR, Tonsgard JH, Ullrich NJ, Allen JC, Rosser TL, Campian JL, et al. Preliminary report of a multicenter, phase 2 study of bevacizumab in children and adults with neurofibromatosis 2 and progressive vestibular schwannomas: An NF clinical trials consortium study. Journal of Clinical Oncology. 2018;**36**(15_suppl):2056-2056. Available from: http://ascopubs.org/doi/10.1200/JCO.2018.36.15_suppl.2056

[31] Wong H-K, Shimizu A, Kirkpatrick ND, Garkavtsev I, Chan AW, di Tomaso E, et al. Merlin/NF2 regulates angiogenesis in schwannomas through a Rac1/semaphorin 3F-dependent mechanism. Neoplasia. 2012;**14**(2):84-94. Available from: http://www.ncbi.nlm.nih.gov/pubmed/22431917

[32] Beltrami S, Kim R, Gordon J. Neurofibromatosis type 2 protein, NF2: An uncoventional cell cycle regulator. Anticancer Research. 2013;**33**(1):1-11. Available from: http://www.ncbi.nlm.nih.gov/pubmed/23267122

[33] Lallemand D, Manent J, Couvelard A, Watilliaux A, Siena M, Chareyre F, et al. Merlin regulates transmembrane receptor accumulation and signaling at the plasma membrane in primary mouse Schwann cells and in human schwannomas. Oncogene. 2009;**28**(6):854-865. Available from: http://www.nature.com/articles/onc2008427

[34] Fraenzer J-T, Pan H, Minimo L, Smith G, Knauer D, Hung G. Overexpression of the NF2 gene inhibits schwannoma cell proliferation through promoting PDGFR degradation. International Journal of Oncology. 2003;**23**(6):1493-1500. Available from: http://www.spandidos-publications.com/10.3892/ijo.23.6.1493

[35] Ammoun S, Flaiz C, Ristic N, Schuldt J, Hanemann CO. Dissecting

and targeting the growth factor-dependent and growth factor-independent extracellular signal-regulated kinase pathway in human Schwannoma. Cancer Research. 2008;**68**(13):5236-5245. Available from: http://www.ncbi.nlm.nih.gov/pubmed/18593924

[36] McClatchey AI, Giovannini M. Membrane organization and tumorigenesis—the NF2 tumor suppressor, Merlin. Genes & Development. 2005;**19**(19):2265-2277. Available from: http://www.ncbi.nlm.nih.gov/pubmed/16204178

[37] Curto M, Cole BK, Lallemand D, Liu C-H, McClatchey AI. Contact-dependent inhibition of EGFR signaling by Nf2/Merlin. The Journal of Cell Biology. 2007;**177**(5):893-903. Available from: http://www.ncbi.nlm.nih.gov/pubmed/17548515

[38] Curto M, Mcclatchey AI. Nf2/Merlin: A coordinator of receptor signalling and intercellular contact. British Journal of Cancer. 2008;**98**:256-262. Available from: www.bjcancer.com

[39] Cole BK, Curto M, Chan AW, McClatchey AI. Localization to the cortical cytoskeleton is necessary for Nf2/merlin-dependent epidermal growth factor receptor silencing. Molecular and Cellular Biology. 2008;**28**(4):1274-1284. Available from: http://www.ncbi.nlm.nih.gov/pubmed/18086884

[40] Hilton DA, Ristic N, Hanemann CO. Activation of ERK, AKT and JNK signalling pathways in human schwannomas *in situ*. Histopathology. 2009;**55**(6):744-749. Available from: http://doi.wiley.com/10.1111/j.1365-2559.2009.03440.x

[41] Jacob A, Lee TX, Neff BA, Miller S, Welling B, Chang L-S. Phosphatidylinositol 3-kinase/AKT pathway activation in human vestibular Schwannoma. Otology & Neurotology. 2008;**29**(1):58-68. Available from: https://insights.ovid.com/crossref?an=00129492-200801000-00013

[42] Petrilli AM, Fernández-Valle C. Role of Merlin/NF2 inactivation in tumor biology. Oncogene. 2016;**35**(5):537-548. Available from: http://www.ncbi.nlm.nih.gov/pubmed/25893302

[43] Bush ML, Oblinger J, Brendel V, Santarelli G, Huang J, Akhmametyeva EM, et al. AR42, a novel histone deacetylase inhibitor, as a potential therapy for vestibular schwannomas and meningiomas. Neuro-Oncology. 2011;**13**(9):983-999. Available from: http://www.ncbi.nlm.nih.gov/pubmed/21778190

[44] Agnihotri S, Gugel I, Remke M, Bornemann A, Pantazis G, Mack SC, et al. Gene-expression profiling elucidates molecular signaling networks that can be therapeutically targeted in vestibular schwannoma. Journal of Neurosurgery. 2014;**121**(6):1434-1445. Available from: http://www.ncbi.nlm.nih.gov/pubmed/25245477

[45] James MF, Han S, Polizzano C, Plotkin SR, Manning BD, Stemmer-Rachamimov AO, et al. NF2/Merlin is a novel negative regulator of mTOR complex 1, and activation of mTORC1 is associated with meningioma and Schwannoma growth. Molecular and Cellular Biology. 2009;**29**(15):4250. Available from: http://www.ncbi.nlm.nih.gov/pubmed/19451225

[46] Jacinto E, Loewith R, Schmidt A, Lin S, Rüegg MA, Hall A, et al. Mammalian TOR complex 2 controls the actin cytoskeleton and is rapamycin insensitive. Nature Cell Biology. 2004;**6**(11):1122-1128. Available from: http://www.ncbi.nlm.nih.gov/pubmed/15467718

[47] Giovannini M, Bonne N-X, Vitte J, Chareyre F, Tanaka K, Adams R, et al. mTORC1 inhibition delays growth of neurofibromatosis type 2 schwannoma. Neuro-Oncology. 2014;**16**(4):493-504. Available from: http://www.ncbi.nlm.nih.gov/pubmed/24414536

[48] Plotkin SR, Merker VL, Halpin C, Jennings D, McKenna MJ, Harris GJ, et al. Bevacizumab for progressive vestibular Schwannoma in Neurofibromatosis type 2. Otology & Neurotology. 2012;**33**(6):1046-1052

[49] Morris KA, Golding JF, Axon PR, Afridi S, Blesing C, Ferner RE, et al. Bevacizumab in neurofibromatosis type 2 (NF2) related vestibular schwannomas: A nationally coordinated approach to delivery and prospective evaluation. Neuro-Oncology Practice. 2016;**3**(4):281-289. Available from: https://academic.oup.com/nop/article/3/4/281/2583805

[50] Hochart A, Gaillard V, Baroncini M, André N, Vannier J-P, Vinchon M, et al. Bevacizumab decreases vestibular schwannomas growth rate in children and teenagers with neurofibromatosis type 2. Journal of Neuro-Oncology. 2015;**124**(2):229-236. Available from: http://link.springer.com/10.1007/s11060-015-1828-8

[51] Baser ME, Mautner V-F, Parry DM, Evans DGR. Methodological issues in longitudinal studies: Vestibular schwannoma growth rates in neurofibromatosis 2. Journal of Medical Genetics. 2005;**42**(12):903-906. Available from: http://www.ncbi.nlm.nih.gov/pubmed/15831594

[52] Nunes FP, Merker VL, Jennings D, Caruso PA, di Tomaso E, Muzikansky A, et al. Bevacizumab treatment for meningiomas in NF2: A retrospective analysis of 15 patients. PLoS One. 2013;**8**(3):e59941. Available from: http://www.ncbi.nlm.nih.gov/pubmed/23555840

[53] Morris KA, Afridi SK, Evans DG, Hensiek AE, McCabe MG, Kellett M, et al. The response of spinal cord ependymomas to bevacizumab in patients with neurofibromatosis type 2. Journal of Neurosurgery. Spine. 2016;**26**(4):474-482

[54] Mukherjee J, Kamnasaran D, Balasubramaniam A, Radovanovic I, Zadeh G, Kiehl T-R, et al. Human Schwannomas express activated platelet-derived growth factor receptors and c-kit and are growth inhibited by Gleevec (Imatinib Mesylate). Cancer Research. 2009;**69**(12):5099-5107. Available from: http://www.ncbi.nlm.nih.gov/pubmed/19509233

[55] Ammoun S, Cunliffe CH, Allen JC, Chiriboga L, Giancotti FG, Zagzag D, et al. ErbB/HER receptor activation and preclinical efficacy of lapatinib in vestibular schwannoma. Neuro-Oncology. 2010;**12**(8):834-843; Available from: https://academic.oup.com/neuro-oncology/article-abstract/12/8/834/1074273

[56] Karajannis MA, Legault G, Hagiwara M, Ballas MS, Brown K, Nusbaum AO, et al. Phase II trial of lapatinib in adult and pediatric patients with neurofibromatosis type 2 and progressive vestibular schwannomas. Neuro-Oncology. 2012;**14**(9):1163-1170. Available from: http://www.ncbi.nlm.nih.gov/pubmed/22844108

[57] Van Gompel JJ, Agazzi S, Carlson ML, Adewumi DA, Hadjipanayis CG, Uhm JH, et al. Congress of Neurological Surgeons systematic review and evidence-based guidelines on emerging therapies for the treatment of patients with vestibular Schwannomas. Neurosurgery. 2018;**82**(2):E52-E54. Available from: http://academic.oup.com/neurosurgery/article/82/2/E52/4764051

[58] Osorio DS, Hu J, Stanek J, Hagiwara M, Wisoff J, Golfinos JG,

et al. MNGO-17 effects of lapatinib on meningiomas in adults with neurofibromatosis type 2 (NF2). Neuro-Oncology. 2015;**17**:v130-v134; Available from: https://www.ncbi.nlm.nih.gov/pmc/articles/PMC4638955/pdf/nov220.16.pdf

[59] Plotkin SR, Halpin C, McKenna MJ, Loeffler JS, Batchelor TT, Barker FG, et al. Erlotinib for progressive vestibular schwannoma in neurofibromatosis 2 patients. Otology & Neurotology. 2010;**31**(7):1135-1143. Available from: http://www.ncbi.nlm.nih.gov/pubmed/20736812

[60] Troutman S, Moleirinho S, Kota S, Nettles K, Fallahi M, Johnson GL, et al. Crizotinib inhibits NF2-associated schwannoma through inhibition of focal adhesion kinase 1. Oncotarget. 2016;**7**(34):54515-54525. Available from: http://www.ncbi.nlm.nih.gov/pubmed/27363027

[61] Poulikakos PI, Xiao G-H, Gallagher R, Jablonski S, Jhanwar SC, Testa JR. Re-expression of the tumor suppressor NF2/merlin inhibits invasiveness in mesothelioma cells and negatively regulates FAK. Oncogene. 2006;**25**(44):5960-5968. Available from: http://www.nature.com/articles/1209587

[62] Fuse MA, Plati SK, Burns SS, Dinh CT, Bracho O, Yan D, et al. Combination therapy with c-met and Src inhibitors induces Caspase-dependent apoptosis of Merlin-deficient Schwann cells and suppresses growth of Schwannoma cells. Molecular Cancer Therapeutics. 2017;**16**(11):2387-2398. Available from: http://www.ncbi.nlm.nih.gov/pubmed/28775147

[63] Dilwali S, Roberts D, Stankovic KM. Interplay between VEGF-A and cMET signaling in human vestibular schwannomas and schwann cells. Cancer Biology & Therapy. 2015;**16**(1):170-175. Available from: http://www.ncbi.nlm.nih.gov/pubmed/25692621

[64] Smith A, Bessler W, Jiang L, Li X, Lu Q, Yuan J, et al. EXTH-13. Reduction of tumor burden and hearing loss with a multiple receptor tyrosine kinase inhibitor brigatinib in a genetically engineered mouse model of neurofibromatosis type 2. Neuro-Oncology. 2018;**20**(suppl_6):vi87-vi87. Available from: https://academic.oup.com/neuro-oncology/article/20/suppl_6/vi87/5154242

[65] James MF, Stivison E, Beauchamp R, Han S, Li H, Wallace MR, et al. Regulation of mTOR complex 2 signaling in Neurofibromatosis 2-deficient target cell types. Molecular Cancer Research. 2012;**10**(5):649-659. Available from: http://www.ncbi.nlm.nih.gov/pubmed/22426462

[66] Goutagny S, Raymond E, Esposito-Farese M, Trunet S, Mawrin C, Bernardeschi D, et al. Phase II study of mTORC1 inhibition by everolimus in neurofibromatosis type 2 patients with growing vestibular schwannomas. Journal of Neuro-Oncology. 2015;**122**:313-320. Available from: http://ctep.cancer.gov

[67] Karajannis MA, Legault G, Hagiwara M, Giancotti FG, Filatov A, Derman A, et al. Phase II study of everolimus in children and adults with neurofibromatosis type 2 and progressive vestibular schwannomas. Neuro-Oncology. 2014;**16**(2):292-297. Available from: https://www.ncbi.nlm.nih.gov/pmc/articles/PMC3895376/pdf/not150.pdf

[68] Goutagny S, Marco G, Michel K. A 4-year phase II study of everolimus in NF2 patients with growing vestibular schwannomas. Journal of Neuro-Oncology. 2017;**133**:443-445. Available from: https://link.springer.com/content/pdf/10.1007%2Fs11060-017-2447-3.pdf

[69] Beauchamp RL, James MF, DeSouza PA, Wagh V, Zhao W-N, Jordan JT, et al. A high-throughput kinome screen reveals serum/glucocorticoid-regulated kinase 1 as a therapeutic target for NF2-deficient meningiomas. Oncotarget. 2015;**6**(19):16981-16997. Available from: http://www.ncbi.nlm.nih.gov/pubmed/26219339

[70] Lin T-Y, Fenger J, Murahari S, Bear MD, Kulp SK, Wang D. et al., AR-42, a novel HDAC inhibitor, exhibits biologic activity against malignant mast cell lines via down-regulation of constitutively activated kit. Blood. 2010;**115**(21):4217-4225; Available from: www.bloodjournal.org

[71] Morrison H, Sperka T, Manent J, Giovannini M, Ponta H, Herrlich P. Merlin/Neurofibromatosis type 2 suppresses growth by inhibiting the activation of Ras and Rac. Cancer Research. 2007;**67**(2):520-527. Available from: http://www.ncbi.nlm.nih.gov/pubmed/17234759

[72] Ammoun S, Ristic N, Matthies C, Hilton DA, Hanemann CO. Targeting ERK1/2 activation and proliferation in human primary schwannoma cells with MEK1/2 inhibitor AZD6244. Neurobiology of Disease. 2010;**37**(1):141-146. Available from: https://www.sciencedirect.com/science/article/pii/S0969996109002691#bib19

Section 4

Cognitive Issues Experienced by Individuals Living with Neurofibromatosis

Chapter 4

Cognitive Issues Experienced by Individuals Living with Neurofibromatosis

Brian S. Potter and Leanne Mendoza

Abstract

In this chapter, we will review cognitive issues faced by individuals living with neurofibromatosis. The chapter will discuss the complicated and sometimes inconsistent cognitive issues and adaptive functioning struggles associated with NF1, NF2, and schwannomatosis. We will review neurocognitive outcomes associated with each of these conditions across the lifespan while focusing on NF1. Specific neurocognitive domains we will review include: intellect, memory, language, nonverbal skills, attention, and executive functions. We will discuss the heterogeneity of the cognitive phenotype for each of these conditions. We will include how associated medical complications such as brain tumor, seizures, and hearing loss can impact neurocognitive outcomes. The chapter will also review the functional consequence of cognitive difficulties including academic struggles, learning disabilities, and decreased quality of life that are sometimes seen in this population.

Keywords: neurofibromatosis, schwannomatosis, cognitive, neurocognitive, learning, lifespan

1. Introduction

Neurofibromatosis is a collection of three distinct autosomal dominant genetic disorders including neurofibromatosis type 1 (NF1), neurofibromatosis type 2 (NF2), and schwannomatosis. Each of these disorders has their own genetic variant, symptoms, and disease course [1]. These disorders are neurocutaneous syndromes, which represent a group of central nervous system (CNS) disorders with simultaneous lesions of other organs such as the skin or eye. One core common symptom among these conditions is that they cause tumors of nerve sheath [2].

In this chapter, we discuss cognitive, academic, and adaptive effects of neurofibromatosis over the course of the lifespan. Through review and synthesis of the extant literature, we summarize what is currently known regarding cognitive sequelae associated with neurofibromatosis and discuss the functional impact with regard to learning, academics, and overall quality of life (QoL). Neurofibromatosis is a multisystem disorder that can cause multiple nerve sheath tumors throughout the body [1]. Each of the three conditions present with their own distinct as well as overlapping symptoms that can have a negative impact on QoL (e.g., chronic pain, bone abnormalities, skin disorders, hearing problems, and learning disabilities) [3, 4]. The presence of benign and malignant tumors, depending on their presentation and treatment regimen, can impact cognitive and developmental functioning [1]. Understanding the functional impact of this disorder is especially crucial in order to improve quality of life throughout the lifespan, as there is no known cure for neurofibromatosis [3]. NF1 is one of the most prevalent and researched genetic disorders. In contrast, prevalence rates of NF2 and Schwannomatosis are much lower, and related research is much more limited. As such, this chapter will focus on the most common of the genetic conditions, NF1.

NF1 is characterized by cutaneous symptoms, including café-au-lait spots, skin neurofibromas, bone abnormalities (e.g., scoliosis), and glial cell tumors (gliomas) [2]. It is associated with a range of developmental and cognitive issues that are present throughout the lifespan. Cognitive and learning problems are the most common complications associated with NF1 [5–7]. In contrast, we did not find any studies that directly investigate the cognitive impact and learning issues of NF2 or Schwannomatosis. This is likely in part because these conditions are less prevalent and believed not to be directly associated with learning issues or academic struggles. That said, these are multisystem conditions that can impact vision and hearing, which can have indirect impact on cognitive skills and learning. Thus, we will discuss the cognitive effects of NF2 and Schwannomatosis indirectly by looking at associated common symptoms of the disorders that can impact cognition. NF2 is defined by bilateral vestibular schwannomas (i.e., benign Schwann cell tumors on the vestibulocochlear nerve), which can cause hearing loss and balance issues [1]. Schwannomatosis is the newest recognized form of neurofibromatosis and is characterized by multiple schwannomas that typically occur in adulthood [1]. The degree of physical/medical phenotypical symptom presentation of each of these conditions is highly variable [1, 3]. Not surprisingly, the cognitive impact of these disorders has been found to be just as variable, which will be discussed more in detail below. At this time, the current literature does not demonstrate to what extent specific cognitive skills are related to each NF phenotype, and it is not yet known whether the presence of predisposing genetic factors for each variant of NF explain this heterogeneity of cognitive outcomes.

2. Neurofibromatosis type 1 (NF1)

Because the phenotypic expression of NF1 is so variable, some individuals living with NF1 are unaware they have the disorder while others are significantly impacted. Additionally, symptoms and signs of NF1 can be fluid and can change in presentation throughout a person's life [8]. In more severe presentations, NF1 can cause physical disfigurement and can be accompanied by significant neurological problems, such as brain tumor and seizures [2]. As noted above, NF1 is a disorder that affects multiple systems in the body, including the brain.

There have been many studies that have investigated the cognitive and learning issues associated with NF1 across age groups throughout the lifespan. One reason that the cognitive and learning struggles associated with NF1 have been well-researched is that NF1 is a single gene disorder (i.e., a mutation of the tumor suppressor gene on chromosome 17), and as such it presents an opportunity to investigate cognitive dysfunction at the molecular and cellular level [9]. The NF1 gene encodes the neurofibromin protein, which serves a vital role in regulating the development of the brain [10]. Brain abnormalities have been detected in magnetic resonance imaging (MRI) studies of those with NF1, such as increased white matter volume, increased subcortical gray matter volume in the thalamus right caudate, decreased cortical gray matter density, T2 hyperintensities (T2H), macrocephaly, and reduced integrity of white matter microstructure [11–13]. Research has also indicated that thalamic T2H as well as volume abnormalities in the corpus callosum, putamen, and amygdala are specifically associated with cognitive deficits in NF1

[11, 14]. Of note, studies looking into the number of T2 spots and how this relates to cognitive impairment have been inconsistently documented [15].

Medical complications that can co-occur with NF1 may lead to or compound cognitive deficits. For example, children with oncological complications of NF1 (e.g., brain tumors) are at risk for long-term cognitive issues as a result of treatment with chemotherapy and/or cranial irradiation [16]. Optic gliomas, tumors that arise from the nerve sheath of the optic nerve, are fairly common in children with NF1 and are sometimes associated with visual impairment, which can impact cognitive skills. The presence of a brain tumor also increases the risk of seizures or additional tumors arising in other areas of the brain [17], which can lead to specific cognitive deficits dependent on the area of the brain it is impacting. NF1 has also been associated with increased rates of other rarer neurological conditions that have known cognitive effects, including cortical dysplasia and hemimegalencephaly, as well as cerebrovascular diseases such as Moyamoya syndrome [17–19].

Just as the severity of phenotypic expression and incidences of medical symptoms are quite variable within those with NF1, the impact on the CNS and subsequent cognitive and academic functioning are significantly heterogeneous. Cognitive and academic weaknesses are some of the most common symptoms in NF1 [5–7]. Cognitive weaknesses can present challenges for the individual, and this has been shown to occur across the lifespan [7]. Findings from studies with very young children have noted that developmental delays and subsequent academic struggles and learning disabilities are pervasive [12, 20]. With regard to investigations with adults and elderly adults, cognitive weaknesses have been noted to be fairly stable over time from childhood [6, 21, 22]. Overall, the level and type of functional impairment may vary depending on what period in life an individual is in (e.g., preschool, school aged, college, working adult, elderly). Across age groups, cognitive issues associated with NF1 have significant associated morbidities, including weaker adaptive skills [15]. Additional consequences of cognitive difficulties associated with NF1 include poorer academic achievement and overall reduced QoL [3].

Below we will provide an in-depth discussion on the cognitive morbidities associated with NF1 as indicated by current research. **Table 1** summarizes specific cognitive domains and findings related to the NF1 population, including overall intellectual ability as well as underlying cognitive functions including language, nonverbal skills, memory, attention, executive functions, academic skills, and adaptive skills.

Studies investigating specific cognitive domains as they relate to NF1 have been wide ranging in their outcomes. Early on, it was believed that in childhood, NF1 was associated with a "nonverbal learning disability" (NLD) profile, a former term for what encompasses deficits in visual–spatial, fine motor, and handwriting abilities in the context of preserved verbal functioning [23]; however, later research challenged this notion with findings indicating that features of NLD are inconsistent among NF1 populations [24, 25]. Additionally, the comorbidity of learning difficulties with these deficits has been found to significantly vary [6, 24]. This is likely in part due to the heterogeneity of the clinical presentation of the condition as well as methodological issues used in research studies, including differences in approaches to cognitive measurement and how learning problems are operationally defined.

Additional studies examining the cognitive outcomes associated with NF1 have led to mixed findings and indicate varying degrees of prevalence of cognitive and academic problems. Hyman et al. [6] noted that these issues were likely due to research design factors, such low sample sizes, lack of controls, subject and control selection, as well as how learning problems are operationally defined. Individual cognitive test sensitivity and measures with overlapping cognitive domains have also been identified as leading to variability [26]. For example, performance on a

Domain	Definition	Common findings
Intellectual ability (IQ)	Summary score of overall cognitive/reasoning ability	Multiple studies suggest IQ to be mildly reduced (IQ ~ 90)
Language	How well a person expresses (including speech) and understands language	Studies have varied. Weaknesses with expressive language and speech are more common than receptive language issues Limited studies in adults.
Nonverbal skills	Visual spatial and fluid reasoning skills	Weaknesses are very common; however, recent studies suggest that findings are confounded by executive function demands inherent in nonverbal measures
Memory	Learning and retention of information	Studies on explicit memory have been variable. Weakness with working memory (short term memory) are common
Attention	Ability to focus, maintain focus on a task	Multiple studies have noted attention problems to be very common. Up to 70% of children demonstrate deficit(s) in one or more aspect of attention
Executive functioning	A collection of higher order skills that assist with complex goal directed behavior	Weaknesses are common. Specific weaknesses with planning/organization and working memory
Academic skills	Skills learned in school that include reading, writing, and mathematics	Weaknesses are very common. Studies vary in prevalence from 20 to 75%, which appears in part to how learning problems are defined
Adaptive skills	Basic skills needed for independent living	Mildly reduced, similar to IQ above

Table 1.
Cognitive domains affected in NF1.

commonly used visuospatial task in the assessment of nonverbal skills in children, the Rey-Osterrieth Complex Figure Test [27], can be undermined by weaknesses in attention and executive functions, as well as motor demands on the measure. Studies have varied in findings related to the prevalence of cognitive issues associated with NF1, though most note that cognitive issues are quite prevalent. Hyman et al. [6] noted that 81% of their sample had moderate to severe cognitive issues in one or more cognitive domains.

2.1 Intellectual ability

Intellectual ability is a cognitive construct that is commonly measured by an Intelligence Quotient (IQ), which represents an individual's performance on an intelligence test relative to similar-aged individuals and culminates performance across verbal and nonverbal problem-solving skills. [28] IQ represents what Charles Spearman (1904) proposed in the early 20th century as the *g* factor, which is thought to contribute to successful performance across various cognitive skills. As such, IQ tests utilize a collection of cognitive tasks to determine a person's overall intellectual functioning. Some of the most commonly used IQ tests are the Wechsler Intelligence Tests, which include various versions of assessments for individuals in preschool through adulthood. Most intelligence tests, like the Wechsler tests, are comprised of verbal and nonverbal reasoning tasks as well as cognitive efficiency tests, including working memory and processing speed. This is particularly the case with the older versions of the Wechsler tests, on which most of the published literature on NF1 is based. IQ scores are typically standard scores with a mean of 100 and a standard deviation of 15.

Numerous studies have investigated IQ in NF1 populations. One of the more consistent cognitive findings in NF1 in children is that overall IQ is slightly lower than the normal population. That is, studies investigating IQ have placed the mean overall IQ approximately 10 points lower than normative sample [6, 29, 30]. This finding has been documented when compared to siblings controlling for environmental influences [30]. Hyman et al. [6] compared cognitive performance of 81 children with NF1 to 49 sibling controls. They found that the NF1 group demonstrated mildly reduced FSIQ with a mean of 90.6 compared to sibling mean of 102.6. Interestingly, this study found no associations between IQ and clinical severity, familial history of NF1, gender or age. Socioeconomic status was the only significant predictor of IQ in NF1 in their sample. Mild delays in IQ have also been noted with very young children, and given that difficulties have been found to be stable across the lifetime, this pattern has been noted in adults as well [14, 31]. In a combined adult and pediatric sample of 103 patients with NF1, Ferner et al. [32] noted an overall mean IQ score of 88.6 [32]. This finding appears to be consistent across cultures. Descheemaeker et al. found the overall IQ to be 89.96 in a Dutch-speaking sample [21]. With regard to elderly adults, there is very limited research investigating NF1; however, one small study noted mild delays in overall intellectual ability [22]. Taken together, these studies provide further support for the lack of progressive decline in IQ over time in NF1. In summary, it appears that NF1 is associated with average but mildly reduced overall IQ, which appears stable over the course of a lifespan.

Despite overall average intelligence, NF1 is associated with greater prevalence of intellectual disability. Intellectual Disability (ID), formerly known as Mental Retardation, is defined in the Diagnostic and Statistical Manual of Mental Disorders, fifth edition (DSM-V) as an IQ approximately two standard deviations below the population mean with associated deficits in adaptive functioning [33]. Studies have varied on findings related to the actual prevalence of ID in NF1 populations. Early studies were believed to have significantly overestimated the prevalence of ID due to methodological issues as well as how ID was defined [5]. The rate of ID in NF1 is believed to be 6–7%, which is much less than what was previously believed, though still two to three times the normative expectation [6]. The prevalence of ID increases if neurological complications (brain tumor, seizures) are not excluded [34].

The overall composite score of the Full-Scale IQ likely masks the underlying subtle cognitive profile of NF1. Nearly 80% of people with NF1 have some cognitive deficit [14]. Thus, recent studies have focused on more discrete cognitive domains which we will discuss more below.

2.2 Language

Verbal skills are a collection of cognitive processes that involves language. Language is commonly divided into expressive and receptive language, which is how well a person uses language to relay their thoughts and ideas (including use of speech) and how a person understands language, respectively.

Weaknesses with aspects of language have been found in populations with NF1. Delays in early language development have been noted children as young as 10 months, which appear to persist [20, 35, 36]. NF1 has been associated with weaknesses with nearly all aspects of language; however, studies have not been consistent [37, 38]. Expressive language problems, especially with speech/articulation, have been more consistently found than deficits with receptive language. Additional speech issues include problems with prosody, overall voice qualify, and aspects of speech sounds [37]. Hyman et al. [6] found that 44% of children with NF1 in their sample received speech-language therapy. Batista et al. [36] assessed central auditory temporal function in children with NF1 and correlated it with the results of language testing. They compared 25 NF1 patients to 22 healthy controls on audiometric and language tasks. They found no problems with peripheral acoustic hearing; however, the NF1 group performed more poorly on the temporal auditory processing task. Weaknesses with phonological skills in children have also been documented in several studies [38–40]. Phonological skills are not only associated with language delays but are also a core component of reading disability, which will be discussed further below. Studies on children have documented further weaknesses with verbal concept formation and comparisons as measured by the Similarities subtest from the Wechsler Intelligence Scales for Children (WISC). These findings were consistent compared to normal population and sibling control group [37, 41]. However, studies with childhood populations have not been consistent, as some studies noted that the differences in language disappear when IQ is controlled for [6, 38]. Verbal fluency has been found to be a relatively preserved cognitive function in children [42, 43]. Available literature on language in adult and elderly adult populations is relatively scarce as most studies in NF1 have been with pediatric populations.

2.3 Nonverbal skills

Nonverbal skills are a collection of visual perceptual, visual spatial, or visual-motor skills. They include visual perception, understanding spatial relations, and ability to integrate information from visual stimulus. Visuospatial (also referred to as visuoperceptual) skills have been found to be impaired in most studies involving children [5, 6, 12, 24, 26, 29, 34]. These studies have noted specific deficits in angulation, visual organization, and object recognition. The findings have been consistent when comparing children to normative sample or sibling control.

Early studies on children with NF1 noted a significant discrepancy between verbal and nonverbal reasoning abilities. Weaknesses were noted with nonverbal reasoning skills, while verbal skills were believed to be preserved [25, 44]. However, several follow-up studies did not find the same discrepancy between verbal IQ and perceptual (nonverbal) IQ [6, 25]. Hyman et al. [6] actually noted a pattern opposite of what was expected, with males with NF1 having weaker verbal than nonverbal reasoning compared to females with NF1. It is now clear that NF1 is condition that can impact a range of cognitive functions not limited to nonverbal reasoning.

In addition to nonverbal reasoning, studies with children and adults suggest weaknesses with many aspects of nonverbal skills including visual perception, visual-motor integration, form discrimination, visual organization [6, 21, 41, 42]. Indeed, weaknesses with aspects of visual spatial skills are common in NF1. However, several studies have not found significant differences between NF1 and controls regarding aspects of nonverbal skills [38, 45, 46]. Van Eylen et al. reviewed studies that directly assessed visuoperceptual and visual spatial functioning of children with NF1 [26]. They argue that the measures used to assess nonverbal skills are likely confounding findings. That is, many tasks that are purported to assess nonverbal skills also require other cognitive domains, most notably executive functions. In their sample, they found that when controlling for executive functions and IQ, performance on nonverbal tasks was not impaired. A similar pattern of weaknesses on nonverbal tasks has been documented in adults [21]. Overall, it appears that NF1 is associated with weaker visual/nonverbal skills; however, there are many confounds to previous studies which temper this conclusion.

2.4 Memory

Memory is our ability to encode, store, and retrieve previously learned information. Neuroscientists have identified many forms of memory, which at a basic level is divided into explicit and implicit memory. Cognitive tests of memory often only assess a small portion of memory functions. Cognitive tests typically focus on working memory and explicit memory. Working memory is our ability to actively hold information in mind for a short duration. It is commonly conceptualized as part of a collection of higher order executive functions.

Cognitive tests assess explicit memory with verbal and visual tests. Studies in both children and adults identifying memory weaknesses in NF1 have been variable, and several studies have not found a significant difference in memory performance than controls [6, 21, 37, 41]. Hyman et al. [6] did not find a significant difference in performance on verbal and visual explicit memory tests in children with NF1 compared to sibling controls. Similarly, Krab et al. [41] did not find a significant difference in NF1 children's performance on verbal or visual memory tasks when compared to children with no learning disabilities, children with specific learning disabilities, and children with general learning disabilities. In contrast, several studies have documented explicit memory weakness in children with NF1 [10, 14, 44, 47]. Bulgheroni et al. [47] assessed visual memory with the Rey Complex Figure Test (RCFT) [48]. They compared 18 children with NF1 to 17 siblings and 18 typically developing children. They found that the children with NF1 performed worse on recall memory, with no difference found regarding recognition memory. This pattern suggests that the NF1 had more difficulty with efficient retrieval rather coding and storing of the information, which is often due how the information was initially organized (an executive function). Overall, studies on explicit memory are mixed.

2.5 Attention

Attention involves of collection of processes that allows a person to engage in certain cognitive processing while ignoring others [51]. Attention is a complex system that has many subcomponents that includes focused attention, sustained attention, divided attention, and selective attention.

Cognitive weakness with attention is very common to children, adolescents, and adults with NF1 [7, 37]. Children with NF1 have frequently been reported to exhibit impaired performance on tasks measuring the ability to sustain and switch attention [6, 52]. These findings appear to be consistent across measures of both visual and auditory sustained attention, as well as divided auditory attention and response inhibition [53]. In a large cohort study of 199 children with NF1, approximately 54% were at risk for inattentive behavior based on parent and teacher ratings [43].

Up to 50% of individuals with NF1 meet diagnostic criteria for attention-deficit hyperactivity disorder (ADHD), [37, 54] and research has indicated that incidence rates of ADHD are much more common in children with NF1 than in immediate family members [55]. Neurocognitive deficits associated with NF1 have been found to be more severe in individuals with comorbid ADHD. While both groups have been found to demonstrate deficits in sustained attention, individuals with NF1 and comorbid ADHD have been indicated to be at higher risk [10]. Reduced attention skills in children with NF1 and ADHD have also been found to negatively impact the ability to process and respond to verbal instructions of increasing complexity, suggesting that receptive language skill development may also be vulnerable in this group as a result of attentional difficulties [10].

The behavioral phenotype of ADHD in NF1 also appears to differ from ADHD in the general population. In a large cohort study by Hyman et al. [6], ADHD co-occurrence in children with NF1 occurred equally in frequency among males and females, which differs from the 3:1 ratio of males to females in the general population [43]. Research suggests that ADHD in NF1 also differs from typical ADHD in that the combined subtype appears to occur at the highest frequency followed by the inattentive subtype, while the hyperactive/impulsive subtype is typically found at the highest rates in children with ADHD alone [56]. Additionally, while clinical symptoms of ADHD in children with NF1 and those diagnosed with ADHD are comparable, differences lie in performance deficits specific to each group such that response inhibition processes have been found to be compromised in ADHD, but not in NF1 when compared to healthy controls, suggesting that response inhibition deficits may be less strong compared to those occurring in ADHD [57]. It has also been suggested that NF1/ADHD is not associated with increased frequency of executive deficits related to behavioral inhibition as it is in the general ADHD population [6]. A study comparing individuals with NF1/ADHD with a group of participants with ADHD and no NF1 found that ADHD symptomatology in NF1 did not exacerbate attention deficits and suggested that ADHD cannot account for all attention impairments in NF1 [57].

Various brain-based characteristics associated with NF1 have been presumed to contribute to the neurocognitive deficits in NF1. For example, increased brain volume due to increased white matter and an enlarged corpus callosum appear to be characteristic of children with NF1 and may interfere with integration and processing of information [56]. Regarding attentional processes specifically, an fMRI study investigating ventral attention networks in the brain found that children with NF1 demonstrated hypoactivation in the temporoparietal junction and the anterior cingulate cortex when compared to typically developing children, which was associated with poorer selective attention and attentional control [58].

The presence of attentional deficits in children with NF1 is associated with even greater risk for poorer performance in other cognitive functions, learning, social skills, and academic achievement [12, 56]. Social outcomes in particular appear to be worse in this group than in children with NF1 only [56]. A study examining face perception in children with NF1 found that sustained attention to faces in a social context is reduced in this population, which may inhibit the processing of socially relevant information needed for successful reciprocal social interactions [59]. Research also suggests that the risk of developing a specific learning disorder is higher in children with NF1 who have a diagnosis of ADHD [6]. As with other domains, it is suggested that while the literature on attentional problems primarily investigates these issues in childhood, these difficulties likely persist into adulthood without treatment.

2.6 Executive functions

Executive functions include a wide range of higher-order cognitive processes that serve goal-directed behaviors, including working memory, planning, organization, inhibition, flexibility. Because executive functioning encompasses a wide range of processes, studies investigating executive functioning in individuals with NF1 vary greatly in terms of the areas of focus and measures used [37]. Of note, many neuropsychological measures of executive function have been found to lack correlation with functional/behavioral ratings of the same constructs when evaluating individuals with NF1, and it has been suggested that Behavior Rating Inventory of Executive Function (BRIEF) rating scale items are more predictive of performance in real-world tasks outside of the structured testing environment [43].

Children with NF1 demonstrate significant impairments across all composite scores on the BRIEF [43, 52]. Differences remained even after controlling for VIQ [43].

Despite this, executive dysfunction has been noted on performance measures as well. Beaussart et al. [50] conducted a meta-analysis of executive functioning in children with NF1. They included 19 studies in their analysis, with a total of 805 children with NF1 and 667 control subjects. They found a moderate effect with executive functions, indicating that children with NF1 had greater overall executive functioning impairments than controls. However, they noted variability in sub-domains of executive functions including cognitive flexibility, planning and problem solving, inhibitory control, and working memory. They found significant effect sizes for each sub-domain, with moderate effect sizes for working memory and planning/organization and small effect sizes for cognitive flexibility and inhibition. Significance remained even after controlling for moderating variables of executive functioning measures, control group composition, IQ, and ADHD.

Weaknesses with working memory in NF1 populations are much more consistent and prevalent than with explicit memory. Several studies have documented verbal and visual working memory weaknesses [10, 14, 49]. Beaussart et al. [50] found a moderate to large effect size for working memory problems. The effect size for verbal working memory was larger than nonverbal working memory. They note that differences in effect size may be due to the psychometric properties of the working memory tasks [50].

Executive function deficits have also been distinguished in NF1 adult populations. In particular, weaknesses in working memory and cognitive flexibility have been noted [21]. Very limited information is known with regard to executive functions in the elderly. Costa de et al. [22] noted working memory weaknesses in this population; however, this study was limited by a very small NF1 group.

2.7 Academic learning

Academic learning entails the use of basic educational skills to be successful in the classroom. This includes reading, writing, and mathematics. Academic learning struggles are one of the most common concerns of parents of children with NF1 [54]. Estimates of learning disabilities have significantly varied between studies. Research has found prevalence rates of learning difficulties to be 20–70% [5, 6, 41]. The variability is in part due to how each study operationalized the definition of "learning disability," as the definition of learning disability has changed over the years. Previously an IQ-academic discrepancy model in which an individual performing much more poorly in an academic skill as compared to his or her overall intelligence level was used to define learning disability; however, this limited definition of a specific learning disability has received increased scrutiny and is rarely used today [60]. Hyman et al. [6] found that 20% of their child sample met the strict definition (discrepancy model) of specific learning disability (SLD), which is double the rate found in the normal population. In contrast, Krab et al. [41] used a different definition that examined "learning efficacy" and found that 75% percent of their sample had learning difficulties based on this definition. This study also noted a connection between disease severity and increase in learning struggles; however, this pattern has not been consistent in other studies. They argue that this is due to the fact that other studies do not systematically measure severity and other methodological issues.

Despite the disagreement in overall prevalence rates of learning struggles, studies have been consistent in that NF1 is associated with significantly higher rate of learning disabilities in children when compared to normative sample and sibling controls [5, 6, 38, 41].

Specific learning disability in the area of reading has been noted in childhood NF1 populations. Weaknesses have been found regarding phonological awareness, word decoding, fluency, and reading comprehension [5, 38, 39, 54]. Cutting and Levine [38] compared four groups that included children without reading difficulties, a reading disability group, an NF1 group without reading disability, and an NF1 group with reading disability. They found that children with NF1 with reading struggles performed similarly as the reading disability group.

Learning struggles in mathematics and written expression in children with NF1 have also been noted. Math difficulties have been noted with computation and application of math concepts [6, 41, 49, 54]. Krab et al. [41] found that 23% of their NF1 sample met the criteria for a specific learning disability in mathematics and 77% demonstrated learning efficiency struggles with mathematics. However, another study did not find learning disability in mathematics [46]. Problems with writing including graphomotor control (penmanship) and spelling have noted as well [49, 61].

2.8 Adaptive skills

Adaptive skills are a collection of functional behaviors needed to effectively meet the demands of our environment. Adaptive functions are often divided into Conceptual skills, Practical skills, and Social skills. The DSM-V notes that adaptive deficits result in the failure to meet developmental and social standard for independent living without support.

Several studies have noted adaptive deficits in children with NF1 [15, 62]. In a cross sectional study of 104 children with NF1, Eby et al. [15] found that 46.5 percent of their sample demonstrated adaptive functioning impairment. They found mild reductions across Conceptual, Social and Practical skill domains. Less is known about the specific adaptive domains that are impacted in adults and elderly adults. While adaptive demands change as individuals develop across the lifespan, it is likely that because cognitive difficulties remain stable with age, adaptive deficits are associated with adults with NF1 as well.

3. NF2 and schwannomatosis

We were unable to locate any studies that directly investigate cognitive weaknesses in NF2 or Schwannomatosis populations. It is likely that this has not been investigated, as these disorders are rarer and typically have less brain involvement. As such, we will discuss the cognitive effects of NF2 and Schwannomatosis with regard to common symptoms associated with these disorders and how these symptoms may impact cognitive functions.

NF2 is defined in part by bilateral vestibular schwannomas [63]. Vestibular schwannomas are nonmalignant tumors that arise from eighth cranial nerve. The vestibular schwannomas can impact hearing, balance, at times vision, and facial weakness [65]. Hearing loss is progressive due to the presence of schwannomas and treatment, and it has been found in 60% of adults and 30% of children with NF2 [65]. Hearing loss can lead to decreased QoL [66] and can impact language development. Hearing loss has also been associated with decreased performance on intellectual and academic skills [67, 68]. Olivier et al. [69] investigated sensorineural hearing loss associated with intellectual and learning struggles in children with brain tumors. They found that children with severe hearing loss demonstrated greater difficulty with reading with weaker phonological skills, processing speed, and reading [69].

Schwannomatosis is clinically distinguished from NF2 by the lack of bilateral vestibular schwannomas and ependymomas [64]. All neurofibromatoses, including NF1, NF2, and schwannomatosis, have schwannomas. Depending on the size and location, schwannomas can also be associated with pain [3]. Chronic pain has been associated with cognitive weaknesses with memory, attention, processing speed, and executive functions [70]. More research is needed to determine the possible cognitive sequalae associated with NF2 and Schwannomatosis. Further research is also warranted to distinguish whether differences in these sequelae exist depending on the age of the individual.

4. Conclusions

Neurofibromatosis is associated with effects on cognitive domains that impact learning, adaptive functioning, and quality of life across the lifespan of individuals affected by these disorders. The three distinct genetic disorders that encompass neurofibromatosis have their own genetic variant, symptoms, and disease course that result in differences in phenotypic expression as well as impact on the brain. While patterns of neurocognitive outcomes vary among and within each disorder, relatively less research has been conducted on those with NF2 and Schwannomatosis as compared to NF1. In particular, more research is needed investigating cognitive sequalae associated with NF2 and Schwannomatosis as these conditions at least indirectly are associated with cognitive weaknesses which can impact overall quality of life, likely from diagnosis through late adulthood.

Within NF1, cognitive deficits are much more common yet highly variable within and between individuals. The heterogeneity of the cognitive outcomes is likely due to a combination of reasons, including genetic factors that have not been adequately elucidated yet, as well as methodological issues. Current research does not yet indicate to what extent differences among each NF phenotype are related to differences in typical cognitive deficits associated with each genetic variant. Common methodological issues in the literature include composition of control groups, evolving/varying definitions of cognitive domains and learning disorders, and limitations inherent in specific cognitive tests. Nonetheless, the current literature indicates that IQ, expressive language, visual spatial and fluid reasoning, and working memory are commonly impacted to some extent. Attention and executive functions appear to also be compromised in individuals with NF1, which are a factor in difficulties in receptive language, memory, academic skills, and adaptive skills. Most studies are focused on children, though existing adult studies suggest that cognitive deficits are present and similar to child studies, likely due to the stability of difficulties over time. Overall, evaluation of cognitive skills in those with neurofibromatosis is important in order to determine the functional impact that potential deficits may have on an individual, especially with regard to academic performance and adaptive functioning. This is especially significant due to the fact that neurofibromatosis is not a curable condition, which necessitates treatment that directly targets cognitive, academic, and adaptive problems directly. Regular monitoring of these individuals with respect to cognitive skills can aid in necessary intervention planning and should occur as early as possible to detect and treat issues that can arise early in development.

Conflict of interest

The authors have no conflict of interest.

Author details

Brian S. Potter* and Leanne Mendoza
St. Jude Children's Research Hospital, Memphis, TN, USA

*Address all correspondence to: brian.potter@stjude.org

References

[1] PlotkinSR,WickA.Neurofibromatosis and Schwannomatosis. Seminars in Neurology. 2018;**38**(1):73-85

[2] Lu-Emerson C, Plotkin SR. The Neurofibromatoses. Part 1: NF1. Reviews in Neurological Diseases. 2009;**6**(2):E47-E53

[3] Vranceanu AM et al. Quality of life among adult patients with neurofibromatosis 1, neurofibromatosis 2 and schwannomatosis: A systematic review of the literature. Journal of Neuro-Oncology. 2013;**114**(3):257-262

[4] Wolters PL et al. Patient-reported outcomes in neurofibromatosis and schwannomatosis clinical trials. Neurology. 2013;**81**(21 Suppl 1):S6-S14

[5] North KN et al. Cognitive function and academic performance in neurofibromatosis. 1: Consensus statement from the NF1 cognitive disorders task force. Neurology. 1997;**48**(4):1121-1127

[6] Hyman SL et al. The nature and frequency of cognitive deficits in children with neurofibromatosis type 1. Neurology. 2005;**65**(7):1037-1044

[7] Walsh KS et al. Behavioral and cognitive outcomes for clinical trials in children with neurofibromatosis type 1. Neurology. 2016;**86**(19):1849-1850

[8] Jett K, Friedman JM. Clinical and genetic aspects of neurofibromatosis 1. Genetics in Medicine. 2010;**12**(1):1-11

[9] Orraca-Castillo M et al. Neurocognitive profiles of learning disabled children with neurofibromatosis type 1. Frontiers in Human Neuroscience. 2014;**8**:386

[10] Monroe CL et al. Dissecting clinical heterogeneity in Neurofibromatosis type 1. Annual Review of Pathology. 2017;**12**:53-74

[11] Huijbregts SC, Loitfelder M, Rombouts SA, Swaab H, Verbist BM, Arkink EB, et al. Cerebral volumetric abnormalities in Neurofibromatosis type 1: Associations with parent ratings of social and attention problems, executive dysfunction, and autistic mannerisms. Journal of Neurodevelopmental Disorders. 2015;**7**:32. DOI: 10.1186/s11689-015-9128-3

[12] Torres Nupan MM, Velez Van Meerbeke A, Lopez Cabra CA, Herrera Gomez PM. Cognitive and behavioral disorders in children with Neurofibromatosis type 1. Frontiers in Pediatrics. 2017;**5**:227

[13] Payne JM, Moharir MD, Webster R, North KN. Brain structure and function in neurofibromatosis type 1: Current concepts and future directions. Journal of Neurology, Neurosurgery & Psychiatry. 2010;**81**(3):304-309

[14] Schutze M et al. Use of machine learning to predict cognitive performance based on brain metabolism in Neurofibromatosis type 1. PLoS One. 2018;**13**(9):e0203520

[15] Eby NS et al. Adaptive functioning in children with neurofibromatosis type 1: Relationship to cognition, behavior, and magnetic resonance imaging. Developmental Medicine and Child Neurology. 2019, 2019;**61**(8):972-978

[16] Vogel AC et al. Neurodevelopmental disorders in children with neurofibromatosis type 1. Developmental Medicine and Child Neurology. 2017;**59**(11):1112-1116

[17] Santoro C et al. Seizures in children with neurofibromatosis type 1: Is neurofibromatosis type 1

enough? Italian Journal of Pediatrics. 2018;**44**(1):41

[18] Pecoraro A, Arehart E, Gallentine W, Radtke R, Smith E, Pizoli C, et al. Epilepsy in neurofibromatosis type 1. Epilepsy & Behavior. 2017;**73**:137-141

[19] Koss M, Scott RM, Irons MB, Smith ER, Ullrich NJ. Moyamoya syndrome associated with neurofibromatosis type 1: Perioperative and long-term outcome after surgical revascularization. Journal of Neurosurgery. Pediatrics. 2013;**11**(4):417-425

[20] Lorenzo J, Barton B, Acosta MT, North K. Mental, motor, and language development of toddlers with Neurofibromatosis type 1. The Journal of Pediatrics. 2011;**158**(4):660-665

[21] Descheemaeker M-J, Plasschaert E, Frijns J-P, Legius E. Neuropsychological profile in adults with neurofibromatosis type 1 compared to a control group: Neuropsychological profile in NF1 adults. Journal of Intellectual Disability Research. 2013;**57**(9):874-886

[22] Costa de S et al. Neuropsychological impairments in elderly Neurofibromatosis type 1 patients. European Journal of Medical Genetics. 2014;**57**(5):216-219

[23] Volden J. Nonverbal learning disability. Handbook of Clinical Neurology. 2013;**111**:245-249

[24] Sally O, Viskochil David H. Cognitive impairment in neurofibromatosis type 1. American Journal of Medical Genetics. 1999;**89**(1):45-52

[25] Mazzocco MMM, Turner JE, Denckla MB, Hofman KJ, Scanlon DC, Vellutino FR. Language and reading deficits associated with Neurofibromatosis type 1: Evidence for a not-so-nonverbal learning disability. Developmental Neuropsychology. 1995;**11**(4):503-522

[26] Van Eylen L et al. Visuoperceptual processing in children with neurofibromatosis type 1: True deficit or artefact? American Journal of Medical Genetics. Part B, Neuropsychiatric Genetics. 2017;**174**(4):342-358

[27] Waber DP, Holmes JM. Assessing children's copy productions of the Rey-Osterrieth complex figure. Journal of Clinical and Experimental Neuropsychology. 1985;**7**(3):264-280

[28] Braaten EB, Norman D. Intelligence (IQ) testing. Pediatrics in Review. 2006;**27**(11):403-408

[29] North K et al. Cognitive function and academic performance in children with neurofibromatosis type 1. Developmental Medicine and Child Neurology. 1995;**37**(5):427-436

[30] Stewart DR et al. Care of adults with neurofibromatosis type 1: A clinical practice resource of the American College of Medical Genetics and Genomics (ACMG). Genetics in Medicine. 2018;**20**(7):671-682

[31] Lorenzo J et al. Developmental trajectories of young children with neurofibromatosis type 1: A longitudinal study from 21 to 40 months of age. The Journal of Pediatrics. 2015;**166**(4):1006-1012.e1001

[32] Ferner RE et al. Intellectual impairment in neurofibromatosis 1. Journal of the Neurological Sciences. 1996;**138**(1-2):125-133

[33] American Psychiatric A et al. Diagnostic and Statistical Manual of Mental Disorders: DSM-5. Arlington, VA: American Psychiatric Association; 2017

[34] Coutinho V et al. Neuropsychological evaluation and parental

assessment of behavioral and motor difficulties in children with neurofibromatosis type 1. Research in Developmental Disabilities. 2016;**48**:220-230

[35] Kolesnik AM et al. Early development of infants with neurofibromatosis type 1: A case series. Molecular Autism. 2017;**8**:62

[36] Batista PB et al. Auditory temporal processing deficits and language disorders in patients with neurofibromatosis type 1. Journal of Communication Disorders. 2014;**48**:18-26

[37] Lehtonen A et al. Behaviour in children with neurofibromatosis type 1: Cognition, executive function, attention, emotion, and social competence. Developmental Medicine and Child Neurology. 2013;**55**(2):111-125

[38] Cutting LE, Levine TM. Cognitive profile of children with neurofibromatosis and reading disabilities. Child Neuropsychology. 2010;**16**(5):417-432

[39] Chaix Y et al. Deficit in phonological processes: A characteristic of the neuropsychological profile of children with NF1. Child Neuropsychology. 2018;**24**(4):558-574

[40] Thompson HL. Evaluation of phonological processing skills of young children with neurofibromatosis type 1. Developmental Medicine and Child Neurology. 2018;**60**(7):642

[41] Krab LC et al. Impact of neurofibromatosis type 1 on school performance. Journal of Child Neurology. 2008;**23**(9):1002-1010

[42] Watt SE et al. An examination of lexical and sublexical reading skills in children with neurofibromatosis type 1. Child Neuropsychology. 2008;**14**(5):401-418

[43] Payne JM et al. Assessment of executive function and attention in children with neurofibromatosis type 1: Relationships between cognitive measures and real-world behavior. Child Neuropsychology. 2011;**17**(4):313-329

[44] Bawden H et al. MRI and nonverbal cognitive deficits in children with neurofibromatosis 1. Journal of Clinical and Experimental Neuropsychology. 1996;**18**(6):784-792

[45] Moore BD 3rd et al. Brain volume in children with neurofibromatosis type 1: Relation to neuropsychological status. Neurology. 2000;**54**(4):914-920

[46] Mazzocco MM. Math learning disability and math LD subtypes: Evidence from studies of Turner syndrome, fragile X syndrome, and neurofibromatosis type 1. Journal of Learning Disabilities. 2001;**34**(6):520-533

[47] Bulgheroni S et al. Visuoperceptual impairment in children with NF1: From early visual processing to procedural strategies. Behavioural Neurology. 2019;**2019**:7146168

[48] Meyers JE, Meyers KR. Rey Complex Figure Test and Recognition Trial. Odessa, Flor: Psychological Assessment Resources; 1995

[49] Billingsley RL et al. Cortical morphology associated with language function in neurofibromatosis, type I. Brain and Language. 2003;**85**(1):125-139

[50] Beaussart M-L et al. Systematic review and meta-analysis of executive functions in preschool and school-age children with neurofibromatosis type 1. Journal of the International Neuropsychological Society. 2018;**24**(9):977-994

[51] Loring DW. INS Dictionary of Neuropsychology. New York, Oxford: Oxford University Press; 1999

[52] Pride N et al. Corpus callosum morphology and its relationship to cognitive function in neurofibromatosis type 1. Journal of Child Neurology. 2010;**25**(7):834-841

[53] Isenberg JC et al. Attention skills in children with neurofibromatosis type 1. Journal of Child Neurology. 2013;**28**(1):45-49

[54] Levine TM et al. Cognitive profile of neurofibromatosis type 1. Seminars in Pediatric Neurology. 2006;**13**(1):8-20

[55] Koth CW et al. The association of neurofibromatosis type 1 and attention deficit hyperactivity disorder. Child Neuropsychology. 2000;**6**(3):185-194

[56] Pride NA et al. The impact of ADHD on the cognitive and academic functioning of children with NF1. Developmental Neuropsychology. 2012;**37**(7):590-600

[57] Lion-Francois L et al. Attention and executive disorders in Neurofibromatosis 1: Comparison between NF1 with ADHD symptomatology (NF1 + ADHD) and ADHD per Se. Journal of Attention Disorders. 6 Jun 2017. DOI: 10.1177/1087054717707579

[58] Pride NA et al. Impaired engagement of the ventral attention system in neurofibromatosis type 1. Brain Imaging and Behavior. 2018;**12**(2):499-508

[59] Lewis AK et al. Attention to faces in social context in children with neurofibromatosis type 1. Developmental Medicine and Child Neurology. 2019;**61**(2):174-180

[60] Fletcher JM, Vaughn S. Response to intervention: Preventing and remediating academic difficulties. Child Development Perspectives. 2009;**3**(1):30-37

[61] Gilboa Y et al. The handwriting performance of children with NF1. Research in Developmental Disabilities. 2010;**31**(4):929-935

[62] Klein-Tasman BP et al. Adaptive behavior in young children with neurofibromatosis type 1. International Journal of Pediatrics. 2013;**2013**:690432

[63] Kresak JL, Walsh M. Neurofibromatosis: A review of NF1, NF2, and Schwannomatosis. Journal of Pediatric Genetics. 2016;**5**(2):98-104

[64] Kehrer-Sawatzki H et al. Phenotypic and genotypic overlap between mosaic NF2 and schwannomatosis in patients with multiple non-intradermal schwannomas. Human Genetics. 2018;**137**(6-7):543-552

[65] North HJD, Lloyd SKW. Hearing rehabilitation in Neurofibromatosis type 2. Advances in Oto-Rhino-Laryngology. 2018;**81**:93-104

[66] Chen J et al. A cerebellopontine angle mouse model for the investigation of tumor biology, hearing, and neurological function in NF2-related vestibular schwannoma. Nature Protocols. 2019;**14**(2):541-555

[67] Farinetti A et al. International consensus (ICON) on audiological assessment of hearing loss in children. European Annals of Otorhinolaryngology, Head and Neck Diseases. 2018;**135**(1s):S41-s48

[68] Grasty MA et al. Hearing loss after cardiac surgery in infancy: An unintended consequence of life-saving care. The Journal of Pediatrics. 2018;**192**:144-151.e141

[69] Olivier TW et al. Cognitive implications of ototoxicity in pediatric patients with Embryonal brain tumors. Journal of Clinical Oncology. 2019;**37**:1566-1575

[70] Nadar MS et al. The cognitive functions in adults with chronic pain: A comparative study. Pain Research & Management. 2016;**2016**:5719380

Section 5

Ocular Findings in Neurofibromatosis

Chapter 5

Ocular Findings in Neurofibromatosis

Hind M. Alkatan, Sawsan S. Bakry and Mohammad A. Alabduljabbar

Abstract

Neurofibromatosis (NF) is an inherited disease affecting multiple systems in the body. The eye is frequently affected in neurofibromatosis, and therefore ocular manifestations play a major role in the diagnosis of NF. This chapter aims to explore the spectrum of ocular manifestations found in neurofibromatosis highlighting the importance of ophthalmic exam in these patients. It will describe various intraocular manifestations involving the iris, lens, and retina. It will be focusing on glaucoma and the pathogenesis behind it in this group of patients. Moreover, periorbital and orbital involvement such as skin neurofibromas and optic nerve gliomas will be discussed along with some of their histopathological findings.

Keywords: neurofibromatosis, glaucoma, cataract, retinal hamartoma, Lisch nodules, choroid, optic nerve, glioma, plexiform neurofibroma, diffuse neurofibroma

1. Introduction

Neurofibromatosis (NF) is an inherited disease affecting multiple systems in the body. It is caused by a genetic mutation affecting cellular growth regulation, therefore resulting in disrupted pathways and formation of multiple tumors in the body. Ocular involvement is an important part of the disease as it may be required for the diagnosis. Although some manifestations are only of diagnostic value such as Lisch nodules, other ocular involvement can be vision threatening like glaucoma and optic nerve gliomas. Therefore, this chapter aims to explore how this disease can affect various structures of the eye and some histopathological changes that may be seen in some.

2. Types of neurofibromatosis

Neurofibromatosis is caused by a gene mutation affecting a tumor suppressor protein resulting in uncontrolled proliferation of neural cells that can involve various parts of the body such as nerves, skin, and eyes. It is classified into two types based on the location of the mutated gene. Neurofibromatosis type 1 (NF-1), also known as von Recklinghausen disease, is caused by a mutation in the gene NF-1 located on chromosome 17. This leads to a dysfunctional tumor suppressor protein known as neurofibromin. As a result, NF-1 manifests as multiple benign tumors in the body such as plexiform neurofibromas, Lisch nodules, and optic nerve gliomas.

Six or more café au lait macules (greatest diameter of >5 mm in prepubertal individuals and > 15 mm in postpubertal individuals)
Two or more neurofibromas of any type or one plexiform neurofibroma
Axillary or inguinal freckling.
Optic glioma
Two or more Lisch nodules (iris hamartomas)
A distinctive osseous lesion (sphenoid dysplasia or tibial pseudarthrosis)
A first degree relative with NF1

Table 1.
Diagnostic criteria for NF1 (two or more must be present).

NF-1 is inherited as autosomal dominant trait but may be sporadic in about 50% of the cases [1]. Ophthalmic manifestations are of diagnostic value in NF. **Table 1** shows the criteria that are used for the diagnosis of NF-1 [2]. Three out of the total seven may involve ocular structures. Therefore, an individual may be diagnosed with NF-1 solely on his ophthalmic exam.

Neurofibromatosis type 2 (NF-2) is caused by a chromosome 22 mutation in the gene encoding for the protein merlin or schwannomin, which is also a tumor suppressor protein. Dysregulation of this gene results in overproduction of Schwann cells. Therefore, the most prominent feature of this disease is bilateral vestibular schwannomas occurring in almost 90% of the patients. It may also affect different structures in the body causing tumors such as optic meningiomas and gliomas. Similar to NF-1, it is inherited in autosomal dominant fashion but may be sporadic [2].

Clinical presentation of both diseases may overlap as they both affect cellular growth of neural tissue. This chapter will be discussing ocular manifestations that are seen in NF highlighting the importance of ophthalmic examination in these patients.

3. Intraocular manifestations

3.1 Iris

Various intraocular conditions have been described in NF, most commonly, iris hamartomas. Iris hamartomas is a hallmark feature in NF-1 and is therefore considered one of the diagnostic criteria. Histologically, Lisch nodules have been described to be a collection of spindle cells that are melanocytic in origin [3]. They usually occur during childhood and increase in size and number with aging. They are typically seen under slit-lamp examination; are described as round elevated nodules within the iris, measuring around 2–3 mm in size; and are brown to yellow in color (**Figure 1**). Lisch nodules are typically bilateral; however, unilateral nodules have been reported previously in some types of NF [4].

3.2 Glaucoma

Glaucoma has been found to occur in about 1 in 300 NF-1 patients [5]. Patients with orbito-facial involvement have been linked to higher rates of glaucoma at 23–50% [6–8]. It was also found that patients with eyelid plexiform neurofibromas have ipsilateral globe enlargement up to 36 mm axial length [6]. Although glaucoma

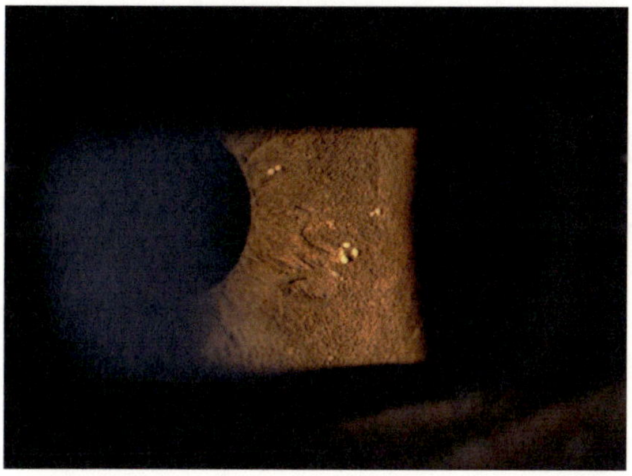

Figure 1.
Slit-lamp photo of an iris showing Lisch nodules in a patient diagnosed with neurofibromatosis.

in NF is not common, it has been studied due to the visual burden it may cause. Various mechanisms have been described in the pathogenesis of glaucoma in these patients. The most commonly described mechanism is the presence of neurofibromas in the angle causing aqueous outflow obstruction [6]. Other suggested processes include secondary angle closure due to the anterior displacement of the peripheral iris by an abnormally thickened ciliary body or developmental anomalies in the angle [7].

Moreover, congenital ectropion uvea has been linked to refractory glaucoma in patients with NF. Histologically, endothelialization of the anterior chamber angle has been observed in these eyes. It has been hypothesized that loss of the NF gene and therefore RAS–RAF–ERK–MAPK pathway activation may be the cause of endothelial overgrowth in these patients [9]. It is difficult to link one mechanism causing glaucoma in NF as most cases are probably multifactorial as described above.

3.3 Lens

Lens opacities are of importance in NF-2 as they may be the first sign to suggest the diagnosis during childhood [10]. NF-2 typically causes posterior subcapsular cataract or cortical cataract and occurs in 60–80% of patients with the disease [10, 11].

3.4 Retina and choroid

Retinal astrocytic hamartomas are benign tumors that usually affect the optic nerve. They clinically resemble a small white mulberry and are mostly linked to tuberous sclerosis but have been reported in NF patients as well. Rarely, those lesions may extend to the peripheral retina and cause devastating complications such as neovascular glaucoma and retinal detachment. Other retinal lesions described in NF patients include combined hamartoma of the retina and retinal pigment epithelium (CHR-RPE) and retinal capillary hemangiomatosis [12–14].

In the past, choroidal involvement was thought to be uncommon in NF patients as it was difficult to visualize subtle changes with fundus examination and conventional angiography. However, with the development of new diagnostic technologies such as optical coherence tomography (OCT), choroidal changes have been found to reach up to 100% of NF patients [15]. Uveal neurofibromatosis has been also demonstrated histopathologically within the choroid (**Figure 2**) [9].

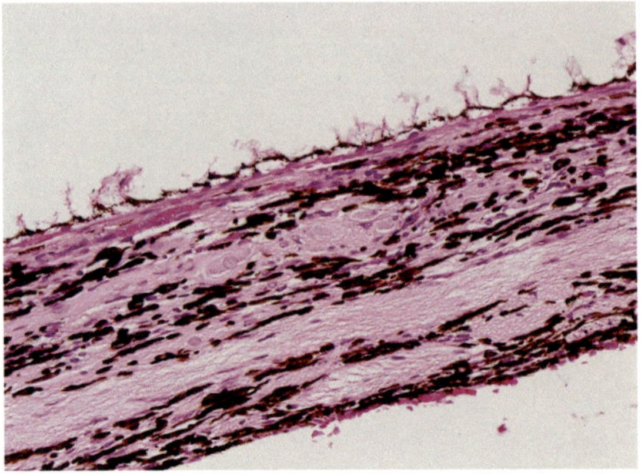

Figure 2.
The choroid in a neurofibroma patient with spindle and ganglion cells (original magnification X400 hematoxylin and eosin).

4. Periocular and orbital manifestations

4.1 Optic pathway glioma

Optic pathway gliomas are low-grade tumors which are classified as WHO grade I pilocytic astrocytomas. They usually occur early in childhood in around 5–25% of NF patients [15]. Although benign, these tumors can cause significant visual loss due to the direct compression of the optic nerve. They may arise anywhere along the optic pathway from the optic nerve to the chiasm and radiation. When those tumors involve the orbit, they may cause unilateral proptosis, strabismus, and decreased vision. Due to the nature of these tumors and the catastrophic consequences they may have, annual screening for all NF patients less than 10 years of age and then every 2 years until the age of 18 years is recommended [16].

4.2 Orbital-periorbital plexiform neurofibroma (OPPN)

One of the most characteristic findings in NF-1 patients and a hallmark of the disease is plexiform neurofibroma. It is a congenital tumor usually unilateral involving the eyelid, orbit, and periorbital area. It starts early in childhood with rapid growth that slows down after puberty. OPPN affects approximately 10% of patients with NF-1, and it carries a risk for malignant transformation in about 10%. It is considered a benign tumor of peripheral nerves with spindle cell proliferation and wavy filamentous pattern of growth (**Figures 3** and **4**). Histologically, they may be composed of mixed diffuse and plexiform types (**Figure 5**) with proliferation of Schwann cells, fibroblasts, and mast cells. Plexiform neurofibromas are similar but are encapsulated with the proliferations being surrounded by perineurium (**Figure 6**). Plexiform neurofibromas are of clinical significance as they are often described clinically as a "bag of worms" and can grow to form bulging masses that can be quiet disfiguring to a patient leading to social embarrassment. They usually cause mechanical ptosis when involving the upper eyelid (**Figure 7**), which may lead to amblyopia in children. Further progression to orbital and periorbital areas lead to proptosis, strabismus, and displacement of the globe. Rarely, plexiform neurofibromas may also involve the conjunctiva of the eye. Sphenoid wing dysplasia can be found in patients with OPPN affecting the same side and usually present with proptosis and pulsatile exophthalmos. Plexiform neurofibroma is a highly recurrent tumor, especially in orbito-facial area and in younger patients [17–19].

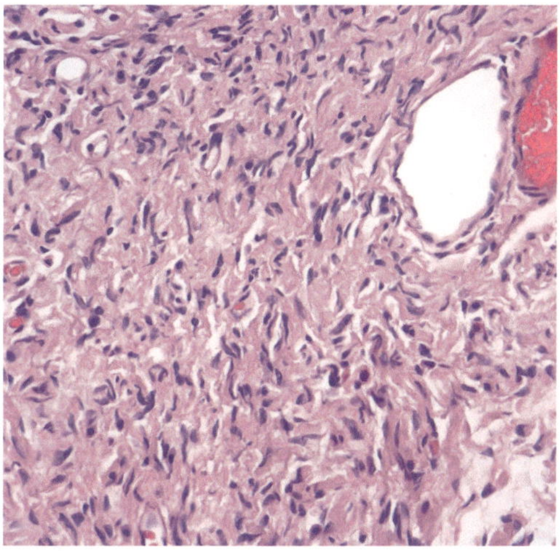

Figure 3.
Neurofibroma of the diffuse type with spindle cell proliferation (original magnification X400 hematoxylin and eosin).

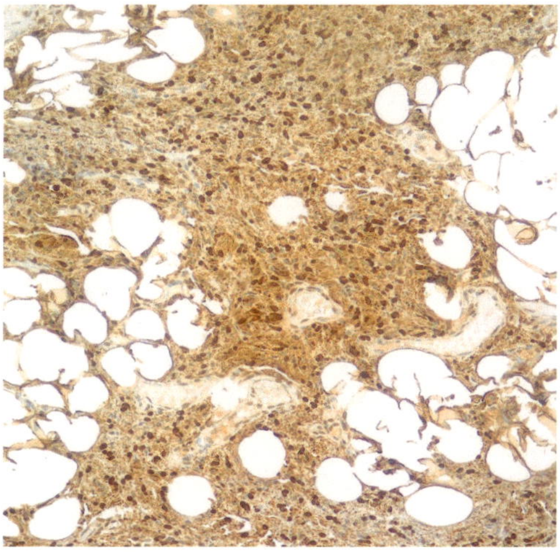

Figure 4.
The same diffuse type of neurofibroma with spindle cells expressing s-100 staining (original magnification X200 S-100).

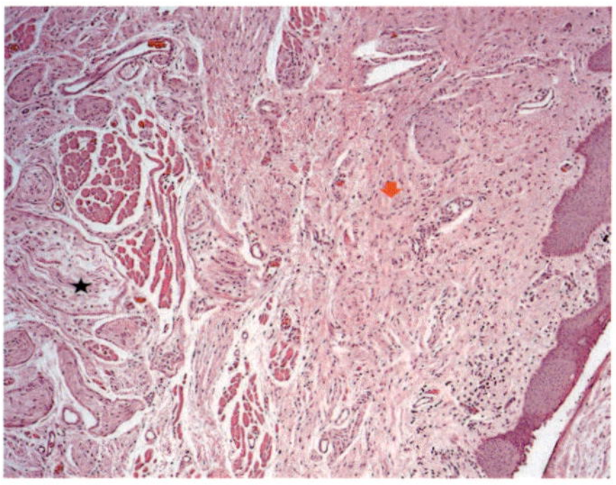

Figure 5.
Mixed plexiform (black star) and diffuse (red arrowhead) neurofibromatosis (original magnification X100 hematoxylin and eosin).

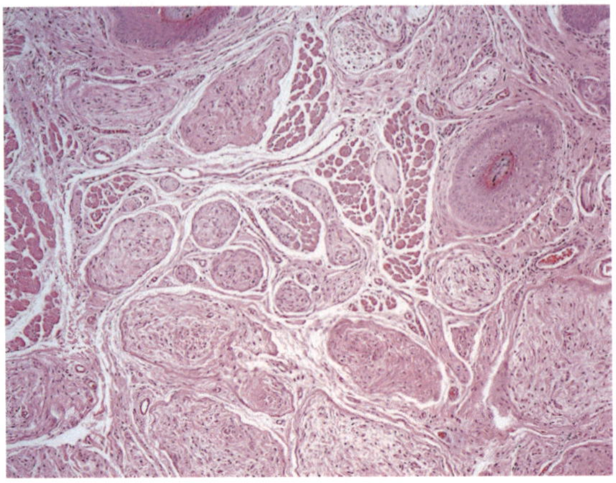

Figure 6.
An area of typical plexiform neurofibroma (original magnification X100 hematoxylin and eosin).

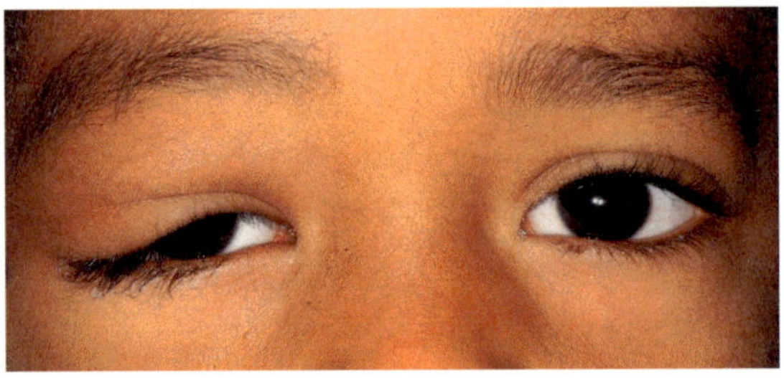

Figure 7.
A child with a plexiform neurofibroma of the right upper eyelid causing significant ptosis that affects the visual axis.

5. Imaging

A high-resolution magnetic resonance imaging (MRI) with and without contrast of the brain and orbits should be performed in all NF-suspected patients to confirm the diagnosis and to monitor for the progression. CT scan should be avoided if possible, because of its radiation and the risk of malignant transformation of neurofibroma [19].

6. Management

Patients with NF need a multidisciplinary team of pediatric ophthalmology, neuro-ophthalmology, oculoplastic surgeon, neuro-oncology, and genetics. All children diagnosed with NF should have regular ophthalmological examinations every 6 months until the age of visual maturation (7 years) to detect and treat amblyopia, glaucoma, or strabismus. Also, serial MRI might be needed. The frequency of examination and imaging should be tailored according to the patient needs and disease progression. Early diagnosis and management of ophthalmic related issues are important and usually treated by supportive methods.

In children, surgical interventions for neurofibroma and its related strabismus should be reserved for severe cosmesis and visually threatening conditions because of its highly recurrent nature. Adults with neurofibroma usually need an aggressive and definitive surgical approach to prevent recurrence with the possibility of several surgeries. The most common indications for surgical debulking are cosmetic, decreased vision, progressive involvement of a vital structure, and functional deficits. Any significant increase in the growth rate of neurofibroma that is unusual for the patient age should be worrisome for malignant transformation [19].

7. Conclusion

In conclusion, neurofibromatosis can affect the eye and ocular adnexa in various ways. It is of importance to recognize ocular involvement in such patients in order to help earlier diagnosis of treatable conditions that can be vision-threatening.

Conflict of interest

The authors declare no conflict of interest.

Author details

Hind M. Alkatan[1*], Sawsan S. Bakry[2] and Mohammad A. Alabduljabbar[3]

1 Departments of Ophthalmology and Pathology, College of Medicine, King Saud University, Riyadh, Saudi Arabia

2 Neurology Department, College of Medicine, King Saud University, Riyadh, Saudi Arabia

3 King Khaled Eye Specialist Hospital, Riyadh, Saudi Arabia

*Address all correspondence to: hindkatan@yahoo.com

References

[1] Thomann K, Marks E, Adamczyk D. Primary Eyecare in Systemic Disease. 2nd ed. New York: McGraw-Hill; 2001

[2] Evans D. Medical management of neurofibromatosis. Paediatrics & Child Health. 2011;**21**(10):459-465

[3] Williamson T, Garner A, Moore A. Structure of Lisch nodules in neurofibromatosis type 1. Ophthalmic Paediatrics and Genetics. 1991;**12**(1):11-17

[4] Adams E, Stewart K, Borges O, Darling T. Multiple, unilateral Lisch nodules in the absence of other manifestations of neurofibromatosis type 1. Case Reports in Ophthalmological Medicine. 2011;**2011**(854784):1-2

[5] Grant W, Walton D. Distinctive gonioscopic findings in glaucoma due to neurofibromatosis. Archives of Ophthalmology. 1968;**79**(2):127-134

[6] Morales J, Chaudhry I, Bosley T. Glaucoma and globe enlargement associated with Neurofibromatosis type 1. Ophthalmology. 2009;**116**(9):1725-1730

[7] Thavikulwat A, Edward D, AlDarrab A, Vajaranant T. Pathophysiology and management of glaucoma associated with phakomatoses. Journal of Neuroscience Research. 2018;**97**(1):57-69

[8] Kahook M, Schuman J, Epstein D. Chandler and Grant's Glaucoma. 5th ed. Baltimore: Williams & Wilkins; 2013

[9] Edward D, Morales J, Bouhenni R, Patil J, Edward P, Cummings T, et al. Congenital ectropion uvea and mechanisms of glaucoma in neurofibromatosis type 1. Ophthalmology. 2012;**119**(7):1485-1494

[10] Kaiser-Kupfer M. The association of posterior capsular lens opacities with bilateral acoustic neuromas in patients with neurofibromatosis type 2. Archives of Ophthalmology. 1989;**107**(4):541

[11] Evans D, Lloyd S, Ramsden R. Neurofibromatosis type 2. Advances in Oto-Rhino-Laryngology. 2011;**70**:91-98

[12] Grant E, Trzupek K, Reiss J, Crow K, Messiaen L, Weleber R. Combined retinal hamartomas leading to the diagnosis of neurofibromatosis type 2. Ophthalmic Genetics. 2008;**29**(3):133-138

[13] Martin K, Rossi V, Ferrucci S, Pian D. Retinal astrocytic hamartoma. Optometry. 2010;**81**(5):221-233

[14] Destro M. Retinal manifestations of neurofibromatosis. Archives of Ophthalmology. 1991;**109**(5):662

[15] Kinori M, Hodgson N, Zeid J. Ophthalmic manifestations in neurofibromatosis type 1. Survey of Ophthalmology. 2017;**63**(4):518-533

[16] Listernick R, Ferner R, Liu G, Gutmann D. Optic pathway gliomas in neurofibromatosis-1: Controversies and recommendations. Annals of Neurology. 2007;**61**(3):189-198

[17] Lewis R, Riccardi V. von Recklinghausen neurofibromatosis. Ophthalmology. 1981;**88**(4):348-354

[18] Arun KP, Thomas Joseph P, Jaishankar HP, Abhinethra MS. Von Recklinghausens disease: A series of four cases with variable expression. Journal of Oral and Maxillofacial

Surgery. 2015;**14**(Suppl 1):161-167. DOI: 10.1007/s12663-012-0399-x

[19] Avery RA, Katowitz JA, Fisher MJ, Heidary G, Dombi E, Packer RJ, et al. Orbital/periorbital plexiform neurofibromas in children with neurofibromatosis type 1: Multidisciplinary recommendations for care. Ophthalmology. 2017;**124**(1):123-132

Section 6

Therapeutic Development in Neurofibromatosis

Chapter 6

Therapeutic Development in Neurofibromatosis

Mina Lobbous and Bruce R. Korf

Abstract

Although neurofibromatosis (NF) was initially recognized in the nineteenth century, only in the past two decades we have witnessed a paradigm shift in therapeutics. This progress is driven by the increasing understanding of the natural history of the NF-associated tumors and understanding of the molecular landscape of these disorders. Multiple clinical trials have been launched evaluating non-surgical treatment modalities and more studies are in the pipeline. Recently, the NF community has adopted standardized endpoints recommended by the Response Evaluation in Neurofibromatosis and Schwannomatosis (REiNS) International Collaboration established in 2011. Such collaborations among academic, regulatory and supporting communities are crucial for providing the infrastructure needed for advancing the therapeutic development in the field of NF.

Keywords: neurofibromatosis type I, neurofibromatosis type II, chemotherapy, radiotherapy, therapeutics, clinical trials, targeted therapy

1. Introduction

The neurofibromatoses are a heterogenous group of familial tumor predisposition syndromes that result from pathogenic variants in tumor suppressor genes leading to dysregulation in various cellular pathways. This dysregulation eventually leads to tumors of the central and peripheral nervous systems as well as multiorgan involvement. The incidence of Neurofibromatosis type 1 (NF1) is approximately 1 in every 2500–3500 births [1], while the incidence of neurofibromatosis type 2 (NF2) is approximately 1 in every 25,000–33,000 births [2]. Schwannomatosis (SWN) has been identified as a distinct entity with different genetic etiology and clinical phenotype from NF2, but it is difficult to assess the precise incidence of this condition. Although the tumors that develop most frequently in NF1, NF2 and SWN are histologically benign, they can cause significant neurologic disabilities and even mortality due to the involvement of the central and peripheral nervous systems. These tumors represent a unique therapeutic challenge due to the heterogeneity in severity and rate of progression among patients and hence novel therapeutic approaches are needed. In this chapter, we will review the recent studies in the field of neurofibromatosis therapeutics along with the collaborative efforts for innovative clinical trial designs.

 IntechOpen

2. The power of collaboration in neurofibromatosis research

The establishment of the NFCTC in 2006 by the Department of Defense was a landmark in the field of NF therapeutics development [3]. The consortium has been in continuous operation since inception. It provides infrastructure, and shared resources across multiple institutions to generate resource-efficient clinical trials. The REiNS working groups are another clear example of the influence of collaboration among NF experts to advance the NF drug development efforts. The Children's Tumor Foundation (CTF) has provided support to the NF community, including efforts to advance research as well as public education and patient support. In 2007, the CTF invested $4 million to launch the Neurofibromatosis Preclinical Consortium (NFPC) to test candidate drug therapies in NF1 and NF2 models. The Neurofibromatosis Therapeutic Acceleration (NTAP) was established as a private philanthropy to accelerate the development of effective therapeutics for pNFs and cNFs. NTAP has partnered with CTF in the evaluation of potential therapeutic agents in animal models of pNFs.

The collaborative efforts among academic, federal regulatory, and private foundations have resulted in early successes in the NF therapeutic development. In February 2018, selumetinib, a MEK1/2 inhibitor co-developed by AstraZenca and Merck&Co, received breakthrough status from the FDA. Selumetinib was granted Orphan Drug Designation based on data from the phase II trial that tested selumetinib in pediatric patients with inoperable pNFs (NCT01362803) [4] and hence, selumetinib may become the first approved drug for NF. This success highlights the power of collaboration, which moved Selumetinib from a repurposed oncology drug to its current clinical success in NF patients. The funders involved for in this "MEK story" are the CTF, the National Institute of Health (NIH), the Congressionally Directed Medical Research Program (CDMRP) through NFCTC, and the NTAP at Johns Hopkins University [5].

3. Therapeutic development in neurofibromatosis type I

Understanding of the pathogenesis and molecular landscape of the NF1-associated tumors has advanced dramatically in recent years. This advancement, along with the continued collaborative approaches across the research community, has fueled therapeutic development efforts against many of the NF1 manifestations. Therapeutic development in NF1 has been tumor-specific, due to the substantial heterogeneity of the development and behavior of NF1-associated tumors across and within patients. Plexiform neurofibromas (pNFs), the source of major morbidity in NF1, has been an area of major focus for therapeutic development, followed by other NF1-associated tumors including cutaneous neurofibromas (cNF), optic pathway gliomas (OPG), and malignant peripheral nerve sheath tumors (MPNST).

3.1 NF1-associated plexiform neurofibroma

Plexiform neurofibromas (pNFs) affect up to 50% of NF1 patients and can involve any peripheral nerve [6, 7]. They occur most commonly in the trunk, followed by the extremities [6]. pNFs tend to grow most rapidly in early childhood and may increase by $\geq$20% per volume per year in young children [8]. Though surgery remains the mainstay for treatment of pNF, complete resection is virtually impossible due to the frequent involvement of adjacent normal tissue, and occasionally critical structures. Moreover, surgical resection is frequently challenging since pNF can cross tissue planes and involve multiple body regions. The most common morbidities leading to surgery are neurologic, disfigurement, and airway involvement [9]. A substantial risk of pNF regrowth after surgical resection has motivated the ongoing research to find non-invasive therapies for pNF.

There are multiple ongoing clinical trials (**Table 1**) targeting pNF which represent a rapid expansion in the pNF therapeutic landscape. Though some of the tested drugs have failed to achieve the primary endpoint, they helped establish the natural history of the growth rates of pNF [10, 11]. The therapeutic development efforts in pNFs had shifted from testing "empirically," usually cytotoxic, agents to agents being supported by well-established transitional studies. The first agent that showed radiographic response was imatinib, with a response rate of 17% [12]. Ras-pathway targeted therapy has been of particular interest, as it provides an opportunity for treating multiple manifestations of NF1 with one drug. For example, Selumetinib, which is a MEK (mitogen-activated protein kinase) inhibitor, has shown activity in pNF and low-grade gliomas (including OPG) associated with NF1 [13].

3.2 NF1-associated gliomas

Optic pathway glioma (OPG) is the most common form of glioma seen in individuals with NF1. While 15–20% of children with NF1 will develop OPG [27, 28] only 30–50% will be symptomatic and one-third will require therapeutic intervention [29]. In those with confirmed decline in visual acuity (VA) or involvement in the hypothalamus, chemotherapy is the mainstay of treatment. First-line chemotherapeutic agents include vincristine and carboplatin [30], while second-line agents include vinblastine [31], vinorelbine [32], and temozolomide [33]. There is a report of four cases of refractory OPG (two sporadic and two NF1-associated OPG) that showed marked improvement in VA following treatment with bevacizumab [34]. These agents rarely restore the premorbid visual acuity and the aim of treatment is usually to stabilize disease and prevent further worsening [35, 36]. Radiotherapy is usually avoided in NF1-associated OPG for concern of secondary tumors [37] and moya moya syndrome [38] Surgical excision of OPG is not feasible due to the tumor location and is usually reserved for instances of complete loss of vision, severe proptosis, or hydrocephalus.

Recently, small molecule inhibitors have been used for refractory OPG in clinical trials (**Table 2**). Among these agents, selumetinib has shown promising results in phase II studies and was proven to be active in recurrent, refractory or progressive NF1-associated pediatric low-grade glioma [39].

Unnecessary cytotoxic therapies for OPG should be avoided, as many OPGs remain asymptomatic and some even regress over time [28]. One of the efforts to standardize the VA assessment in clinical trials for NF1-associated OPG is through using optic coherence tomography (OCT) [40, 41]. OCT provides an objective assessment of the retinal nerve fiber layer thickness. OCT is a noninvasive tool to monitor children with OPG in whom, especially the youngest ones, traditional methods of VA assessment is challenging [42]. Another objective noninvasive tool to asses VA in NF1-associated OPG is automated tractography of the optic radiation that was validated in a recent study [43].

A retrospective study that analyzed the clinical and pathological features of gliomas in 100 individuals with NF1 emphasized the wide histologic spectrum of gliomas in those with NF1 [44]. Indeed, individuals with NF1 have an increased risk of malignant gliomas compared with the general population [45], but there are confounding reports on glioblastoma prognosis in those with NF1 vs. cases without NF1 [46, 47]. A recent study analyzed the molecular landscape of gliomas in NF1 and showed that 50% of low-grade gliomas displayed an immune signature, T-lymphocytic infiltrate, and increased neoantigen load [48], findings that may influence future clinical trials in NF1-associated gliomas.

Drug	Target	Phase	Age (y)	Endpoints	Results
Thalidomide [14]	Angiogenesis	I	>5	ORR	Completed/unclear benefit
Sirolimus [15] NCT00634270	mTOR	II	>3	3D ORR, TTP	Modest increase in TTP, no objective response
Sorafenib [16] NCT00727233	Raf kinase, c-kit, PDGF, VEGFR2,3	I	3–18	3D ORR	Intolerable, decrease in QOL due to pain, no objective response
Pirfenidone [17, 18] NCT00076102	Fibroblast proliferation	I, II	3–21	3D ORR	Completed, no objective response
Cediranib NCT00326872	VEGFR-1, -2, -3	II	≥18	3D ORR	Terminated due to slow accrual
Tipifarnib [19] NCT00021541	Farnesyl transferase	I, II	3–25	TTP, 3D ORR	Completed, No difference in TTP
PEG-Interferon alpha 2b [20, 21] NCT00396019	Immune, angiogenesis	I, II	18 months–21 years in phase II	TTP, 3D ORR	Doubled TTP, 3D ORR less than 20%
Vinblastine/Methotrexate NCT00030264	Cytotoxic	II	≤25	TTP	Completed, pending results
Celecoxib; PEG-Interferon alpha 2b NCT00846430	Immune, angiogenesis	II	2–30	Symptoms improvement, ORR	Active, not recruiting
Nilotinib NCT01275586	BCR-ABL, PDGFR, c-kit	Pilot	≥18	RECIST,3D ORR	Completed
Everolimus [22] NCT01412892	mTOR	II	18–60	3D ORR	Completed, no objective response
Everolimus NCT01365468	mTOR	II	>10	3D ORR, TTP	Terminated due to slow accrual
Imatinib [23] NCT01673009	c-kit, PDGFR	II	3–65	RECIST, 3D ORR	17% 3D ORR

Drug	Target	Phase	Age (y)	Endpoints	Results
Sunitinib NCT01402817	PDGFR, VEGFR, c-kit	II	3–65	3D ORR	Terminated (1 patient died)
Pexidartinib [24] NCT02390752	c-kit, FLT3, CSF1R	I, II	3–31	ORR	Recruiting
Cabozantinib NCT02101736	RET, c-MET, VEGFR	II	≥3	3D ORR	Recruiting
Trametinib NCT02124772	MEK	I	1 month–17 years	PK, PD, toxicity	Recruiting
PD-0325901 [25] NCT02096471	MEK	II	≥16	3D ORR	Completed, 42% 3D ORR
Selumetinib [26] NCT01362803	MEK	I, II	2–18	3D ORR	Active, not recruiting, 71% 3D ORR
Selumetinib NCT02407405	MEK	II	≥18	3D ORR	Recruiting
Binimetinib NCT03231306	MEK	II	≥1	3D ORR	Recruiting
Selumetinib (intermittent dosing) NCT03326388	MEK	I, II	3–18	Toxicity, 3D ORR	Active, not recruiting
Trametinib NCT03363217	MEK	II	1 month–25 years	3D ORR, TTP RECIST	Recruiting
Imatinib (in pNF with airway involvement) NCT03688568	c-kit, PDGFR	II	6 months–12 years	Sleep study/PFT, 3D ORR	Recruiting

Abbreviations: 3D ORR, volumetric objective radiographic response; BCR-ABL, fusion gene of breakpoint cluster region and Abl1; c-kit, kit ligand or stem cell factor; c-MET, MET proton-oncogene; CSF1R, colony stimulating factor 1 receptor; FLT3, Fms-like tyrosine kinase 11; MEK, mitogen activated protein kinas; mTOR, mammalian target of rapamycin; PD, pharmacodynamic; PDGFR platelet-derived growth factor; PFT, pulmonary function test; PK, pharmacokinetics; RECIST, Response Evaluation Criteria In Solid Tumors; RET, rearranged during transfection proto-oncogene; TTP, time to progression; VEGFR vascular endothelial growth factor receptor; ORR, objective response rate.

Table 1.
Clinical trials for neurofibromatosis type 1-associated plexiform neurofibromas.

Drug	Target	Phase	Age	Endpoints	Status
Vinblastine +/– Bevacizumab NCT02840409	Cytotoxic/VEGF	II	6 months–18 years	Response rate, OS, PFS, visual outcome measures, OCT	Recruiting
Pegylated interferon NCT02343224	Tumor microenvironment	II	3–18 years	Response rate	Recruiting
Pomalidomide NCT02415153	Angiogenesis/ immunomodulation	I	3–20 years	Toxicity, MTD	Active, not recruiting
Lenalidomide NCT01553149	Angiogenesis/ immunomodulation	II	0–21 years	Response rate	Active, not recruiting
Everolimus (RAD0001) NCT01158651	mTOR	II	1–21 years	Response rate	Active, not recruiting
Binimetinib (MEK162) NCT02285439	MEK	I/II	1–18 years	MTD, response rate	Recruiting
Binimetinib (MEK162) NCT01885195	MEK	II	Older than 18 years	Response rate	Completed (pending results)
Selumetinib NCT01089101	MEK	I/II	3–21 years	Safety, MTD, Response rate	Recruiting

Abbreviations: MEK, mitogen-activated protein kinase; mTOR, mammalian target of rapamycin; VEGF, vascular endothelial growth factor.

Table 2.
Clinical trials for optic pathway gliomas (OPG) and other gliomas associated with neurofibromatosis type 1.

3.3 NF1-associated malignant peripheral nerve sheath tumors

Malignant peripheral nerve sheath tumors (MPNSTs) are rare high-grade sarcomas with poor prognosis [49]. MPNSTs occur more frequently in those with NF1 compared with the general population, with a lifetime risk of 8–13% [50]. Several studies have not shown a significant difference in the molecular landscape between sporadic and NF1-associated MPNSTs [51, 52]. FDG-PET remains the gold standard noninvasive diagnostic tool for MPNSTs, with 89–100% sensitivity and 72–95 specificity [53, 54]. Surgical resection with negative margins is the mainstay of treatment [55], though that is not usually feasible. Use of adjuvant radiotherapy to induce local control in MPSNTs failed to show improvement in overall survival in NF1-associated MPNSTs [56].

There are limited chemotherapeutic options, including agents like doxorubicin, and ifosfamide [57, 58]. A phase II study of bevacizumab and everolimus that enrolled 25 individuals (17 had NF1-associated MPNST) did not show a clinical benefit (defined as complete response, partial response or stable disease for ≥4 months) [59]. Although preclinical studies showed EGFR amplification in MPSNT [60], EGFR inhibitors did not show clinical activity against MPNST in clinical trials. A few studies have been conducted in sarcomas using targeted therapy, and these have not shown clinical activity; tested drugs included imatinib [61], dasatinib [62], sorafenib [63], and erlotinib [64]. These negative studies emphasize the importance of developing xenografts to explore new therapeutic targets and explore pathways of interest like the NF1/P53-mutant transgenic MPNST model [65–67].

Combined targeted therapy has been used to exploit cellular vulnerabilities of cancer cells, as in RAS-driven tumors which are refractory to conventional therapies. A preclinical study has shown dramatic tumor shrinkage in a transgenic MPNST mouse model in response to combined HSP90 and mTOR inhibition [68]. This promising preclinical work had led to a phase I/II study of gantespib, a novel injectable inhibitor of HSP90 and the mTOR inhibitor, sirolimus. The study enrolled 20 participants (NCT02008877) and results are pending [69]. Another novel approach undergoing phase I study utilizes the oncolytic potential of the genetically engineered injectable measles virus Edmonston vaccine strain (MVEdm) that encodes thyroid sodium iodide symporter [70] (**Table 3**).

3.4 NF1-associated cutaneous neurofibromas

Cutaneous neurofibromas (cNFs) are among the most common manifestations in NF1, affecting about 99% of patients with NF1 [71]. cNFs are unlikely to undergo malignant transformation or to cause fatal complications or severe neurologic disability. Nevertheless, cNFs are considered one of the greatest concerns in patients, especially adults, with NF1. These concerns are mainly due to disfigurement and dysesthesia, causing substantial psychological distress and negative body image perception [72]. There is immense variability in cNF among patients with NF1 with respect to size, location, age at first presentation, associated symptoms, and number. These factors affect the therapeutic approach to cNFs and emphasize the need for reproducible and reliable endpoints to ensure clinical success for tested agents.

Drug	Target	Phase	Age (years)	Endpoints	Status
EGFR806 CAR-T cell NCT03618381	Immunotherapy	I	1–26	Toxicity	Recruiting
Selumetinib and Sirolimus NCT03433183	MEK and mTOR	II	≥12	CBR, PFS, OS	Active, not recruiting
Injectable MVEdm vaccine strain NCT02700230	Oncolytic virotherapy	I	≥18	Toxicity, MTD, ORR	Recruiting
Pazopanib vs. Sapanisertib NCT02601209	PDGFR, VEGFR, c-kit (Pazopanib), TORC1&2 (Sapanisertib)	I (Sapanisertib), II	≥18	MTD, PFS, ORR	Active, not recruiting
Lorvotuzumab mertansine NCT02452554	CD-56 antibody	II	1–30	RECIST	Active, not recruiting
Pexidartinib and Sirolimus NCT02584647	c-kit, FLT3, CSF1R, mTOR	II	≥18	PFS, OS	Recruiting

Abbreviations: CBR, clinical benefit rate; c-kit, kit ligand or stem cell factor; c-MET, MET proton-oncogene; CSF1R, colony stimulating factor 1 receptor; FLT3, Fms-like tyrosine kinase 11; MEK, mitogen activated protein kinas; MTD, maximum tolerated dose; MVEdm; measles virus edmonston vaccine strain, OS, overall survival; PDGFR platelet-derived growth factor; PFS, progression free survival; RECIST, Response Evaluation Criteria In Solid Tumors; TORC, mammalian target of rapamycin complex; TTP, time to progression; VEGFR vascular endothelial growth factor receptor; ORR, objective response rate.

Table 3.
Clinical trials for malignant peripheral nerve sheath tumors in neurofibromatosis type 1.

Clinical management for cNF involves surveillance or procedure-based therapy. Conventional surgical resection promotes complete removal of the lesion, but there are obstacles, including limited number of lesions that can be treated in a single session and the scarring that may be induced by surgical resection. Other alternatives include electrodessication, which remove cNFs through dehydration and denaturation [73]. This allows for removal of large numbers (up to thousands) of cNFs in one session, but it requires general anesthesia and may cause scarring and pigmentation changes. A retrospective study of 106 individuals with multiple, small cNFs treated with CO_2 laser ablation reported >90% patient satisfaction, yet a local infection rate was reported to be 15% [74]. Other procedure-based therapies reported in cNFs are laser photocoagulation [75] and radiofrequency ablation [76]. Another approach using local drug/device combinations is the photodynamic therapy (PDT), which is being tested in different cancers [77]. PDT in cNFs studies use a photosensitizer, 5-amino-levulinic acid, plus illumination with red light. PDT was evaluated in phase I study (NCT01682811) and a phase II study (NCT02728388) is active in a single US institution.

One of the early efforts for treatment of cNFs and their associated symptoms used ketotifen [78]. Ketotifen is a histamine 1 receptor blocker which facilitates mast cell stabilization and; its use in NF1 is based on the finding of abundant mast cells in neurofibromas. Improvement in pain and pruritis has been reported, but objective tumor shrinkage has not been documented. Three drugs have been tested in cNFs using local therapeutic approaches; the first was ranibizumab, a vascular endothelial growth factor monoclonal antibody, which was injected intralesionally (NCT00657202). The overall effect of the treatment was minimal and the variability in the tumor volume assessment (measured by a caliper) limited the interpretation of the data. The second agent was topical imiquimod, which showed minimal efficacy in tumor shrinkage compared to baseline volume (measured by a caliper) (NCT00865644). The third agent was topical rapamycin, an mTOR inhibitor, which was initially tested in Tuberous Sclerosis Complex (TSC)-associated angiofibromas (NCT01031901) [79]. The study enrolled 52 patients with TSC and NF1 and data are expected.

Due to the relatively benign histology of cNFs and the likely need for long term therapy, there are special considerations pertaining to cNF drug development [80]. The safety profile of tested drugs is a major concern to physicians, regulators, patients and their caregiver. Also, the route of administration and cost are important considerations, as individuals with cNF are more likely to require treatment (either medication or intervention) for an extended period of time. The variant phenotype among affected persons, demographic differences, and the goal of treatment are important factor determining the type and timing of treatment.

The above-mentioned considerations, especially the safety profile, make oral systemic therapies preferable for individuals with a heavy tumor burden. Everolimus, an oral mTOR inhibitor, was evaluated in a phase II study of disfiguring cNF associated with NF1 (NCT02334902). The study enrolled 22 patients and used photographic measurement of selected lesion to assess surface volume. While 5/22 patients withdrew due to adverse events, a very modest effect was reported in <20% of the participants [81]. Due to the promising results of using targeted therapied against MEK, selumetinib is being studied in NF1-associated cNFs (NCT02839720). The study is a phase II, multi-institutional, open label study with the primary outcome measure being the change in the size of cNFs assessed by digital photography and caliper measurements.

The Clinical Trial Design and Development REiNS subgroup, involving experts from different settings, has presented the priorities and challenges associated with conducting clinical trials targeting cNF in NF1 [82]. The subgroup members reviewed key topics like natural history, assessment methods, functional endpoints, safety, and development strategies. One of the most important topics, which pose a major challenge in cNF clinical trials, is the measurement of outcomes. Methods of measurement that have been used include calipers, digital and volume photography, ultrasound, and MRI. The subgroup members support considering clinically meaningful measures of effectiveness in interpreting changes in tumor size or number. Tumor size reduction that correlates with improved pain control or discomfort is more clinically meaningful than the crude number or size of the tumors. New approaches, such as high-frequency ultrasound or optical coherence tomography, may be able to address some of the limitations of the conventional methods like MRI, photography or caliper measurement. These new approaches need to be validated through additional studies. The subgroup members recommend several key factors when designing clinical trials on cNF, including timing to initiate intervention, eligibility criteria to ensure diversity, mechanism of the intervention, route of administration, safety monitoring, and regulatory considerations.

4. Therapeutic development in neurofibromatosis type 2

NF2 is an autosomal dominant disorder that affects the central and peripheral nervous systems. NF2 has an estimated incidence of 1 in 25,000–33,000 births, making it far less common than NF1 [83]. Vestibular schwannomas (VS) are considered the hallmark of NF2, and bilateral VS fulfill the clinical diagnosis of definite NF2 [84]. The average age at diagnosis in NF2-associated VS is about 27 years [85]; diagnosis in childhood predicts a severe phenotype and unfavorable prognosis [86]. Though VS are slowly progressive tumors, they can cause significant neurologic disability, including hearing loss and eventually deafness, balance problems, and brain stem compression [87]. The other common tumor associated with NF2 is meningioma, which is the most common intracranial tumor worldwide. Up to half of individuals with NF2 develop meningiomas [88], and despite benign histology, they may lead to a shortened life expectancy [89].

The loss of the tumor suppressor protein merlin in NF2 leads to activation of prosurvival pathways via RAS modulation. Hence, NF2 shares many of the same targets identified in NF1. Merlin is absent not only in NF2-associated VS, but also in sporadic VS [90]. This observation is important as it may point to a shared therapeutic pathway between NF2-associated VS and sporadic VS [91].

Though surgery remains the mainstay of treatment in sporadic VS, or stereotactic radiosurgery (SRS) for tumors <3 cm [92], these approaches have proved to be less efficacious in NF2-associated VS, with high rate of complications, including facial nerve weakness, hearing loss, and headache [93, 94]. Moreover, there are growing concerns about utilizing radiation therapy in NF2 due to risk of late malignant transformation [95]. Some of the challenges that face NF2 clinical trials are the substantial variability in disease severity across individuals with NF2, the lack of clear association between the rate of VS growth and the rate of hearing loss, and the variable growth rates between the right and the left VS in same patient [96]. A prospective study that highlighted the lack of correlation between VS size or growth rate and rate of hearing loss was published in 2014 and included 120 individuals with NF2-associated VS (total of 200 VS) [97]. The investigators used word recognition score (WRS) as an objective measurement for hearing decline and defined radiographic tumor growth as ≥20% increase in tumor volume compared with baseline. The study showed that the mean rate of hearing decline from diagnosis was 5% at 1 year and 16% at 3 years, while the rate of VS tumor graphic progression was 31% at 1 year and 79% at 3 years. The median time to progression

(14 months) was significantly shorter than the median time to hearing decline (62 months) [93]. This study, along with prior reports, elucidated the natural history of individuals with NF2 to help to determine the most appropriate timing for intervention [81, 83, 98].

Clinical trials for NF2 have been focused on vestibular schwannomas, since loss of hearing is often the most pressing concern in individuals with NF2. A group of 36 international researchers, physicians, representatives from the pharmaceutical industry, and patient advocates held a workshop to provide consensus recommendations to accelerate clinical trials progress in NF2 [99]. The group provided recommendations on participant selection, clinically meaningful and feasible endpoints, the clinical trials models most appropriate for NF2, and candidate therapeutic agents for NF2.

Different cellular pathways have been targeted in clinical trials for NF2-associated tumors (**Table 4**), with mixed responses. One of the most promising agents used in NF2 is bevacizumab, which was initially given on a compassionate use basis for adults with NF2-associated VS with severe disability [100, 101]. In these reports, 6 of 10 participants had ≥20% reduction in tumor volume and significantly improved hearing. The promising results led to designing two phase II clinical trials using bevacizumab in persons with NF2 who suffered from progressive hearing loss. A preliminary report from one of these 2 trials that enrolled 22 participants showed that the overall hearing and radiographic response rates were 41 and 23% respectively, though pediatric participants appeared to benefit less compared to adults (NCT01767792) [102]. Bevacizumab was used in a dose of 10 mg/kg every 2 weeks for 6 months, followed by 5 mg/kg every 3 weeks for 18 months; this regimen was well tolerated.

Drug	**Target**	**Phase**	**Age (years)**	**Endpoints**	**Status**
Everolimus [104] NCT01419639	mTOR	II	≥3	VS: 15% volume reductions	No RR
Everolimus [105] NCT01490476	mTOR	II	≥15	VS: volume reduction	No RR
Everolimus NCT01345136	mTOR	II	16–65	VS: volume reduction	Active, not recruiting
Everolimus NCT01880749	mTOR	Early phase I	≥18	VS and MEN: tumor PK, molecular analysis	Active, not recruiting
Lapatinib [106] NCT00973739	EGFR/ErBb2	II	4–80	VS: 15% volume reduction	23.5% RR
Lapatinib NCT00863122	EGFR/ErBb2	Early phase I	≥18	VS: tumor PK, molecular analysis	Completed, pending results
Axitinib NCT02129647	VEGF, c-kit, PDGFR	II	≥18	VS: 20% volume reduction	Active, not recruiting
Nilotinib NCT01201538	PDGF, c-kit	II	≥18	VS: 20% volume reduction	Terminated
PTC 299 NCT00911248	VEGF	II	≥18	VS: Tumor volume or WRS	Terminated
Endostatin NCT02104323	Anti-angiogenic	II	16–30	Tumor volume	Completed, pending results

Drug	Target	Phase	Age (years)	Endpoints	Status
AR-42 NCT02104323	HDAC	Early phase I	≥18	VS and MEN: tumor PK, molecular analysis	Active, not recruiting
Bevacizumab [107] NCT01207687	VEGF	II	≥12	VS: hearing response measured by WRS	Completed, hearing response 36%
Bevacizumab [102] NCT01767792	VEGF	II	≥12	VS: hearing response measured by WRS	Active, not recruiting, hearing response 41%, RR 23%
Acetylsalicylic acid NCT03079999	Antiplatelet, anti-inflammatory	II, randomized, placebo-control	≥12	VS: PFS	Active
Vistusertib (AZD2014) NCT02831257	mTORC1, mTORC2	II	≥18	MEN: RR using volumetric MRI	Active, not recruiting
Selumetinib NCT03095248	MEK	II	3–45	VS, MEN, and ependymoma: hearing response measured by WRS, RR	Active

Abbreviations: c-kit, kit ligand or stem cell factor; EGFR/ErBb2, epidermal growth factor reception; HDAC, histone deacetylase; MEK, mitogen activated protein kinas; MEN, meningioma; mTOR, mammalian target of rapamycin; mTORC, mammalian target of rapamycin complex; PDGFR platelet-derived growth factor; PFS, progression-free survival; PK, pharmacokinetics; VEGF, vascular endothelial growth factor; RR, radiographic response; VS. vestibular schwannoma; WRS, word recognition score.

Table 4.
Clinical trials in Neurofibromatosis type 2-associated vestibular schwannomas and meningiomas.

NF2 shares many of the same targets identified in NF1; hence, some of the therapeutic agents tested in NF1 are being tested in NF2, including everolimus (NCT01345136), sorafenib, and selumetinib (NCT03095248). The dual mTROC1 and mTORC2 inhibitor, vistusertib (AZD2014), is used in a phase II study for NF2 patients with progressive or symptomatic meningiomas (NCT02831257). While the primary outcome for this study is the radiographic response rate for meningioma using volumetric MRI scans, the secondary outcomes include response assessment for VS and non-target meningioma using volumetric MRI. The NFCTC has approved using crizotinib, a MET and ALK inhibitor, in a phase II study for children and adults with NF2-associated progressive VS. There are promising preclinical studies identifying crizotinib as a potent inhibitor of NF2-null Schwann cell proliferation in vitro and tumor growth in vivo [103]. The goal for these clinical trials is to assess the hearing response rate as a clinically meaningful endpoint and to assess tolerability and long term effects of the tested agents, as well as identify biomarkers that can predict outcomes.

5. Therapeutic development in Schwannomatosis

Schwannomatosis (SWN), as the name implies, is characterized by the development of multiple peripheral nerve schwannomas, without concomitant involvement of the vestibular nerve, and, less commonly, meningiomas [108–110]. Since the schwannoma is the most common tumor in NF2 and SWN, there can be overlap between the two syndromes. SWN is a distinct entity with different clinical phenotype and genetic etiology from NF2. Germline mutations in SMARCB1 and LZTR1, both tumor suppressor genes, have been identified in SWN [111–113]. Unlike NF1 and NF2, pain is the most common symptom reported by individuals affected with SWN, with 68% reporting chronic pain in SWN in a retrospective study [114].

Surgical resection is considered the treatment of choice for symptomatic schwannomas for pain relief, though local recurrence is not uncommon. Patients usually require multiple surgical resections due to pain, focal neurologic deficits, or myelopathy [113]. Radiotherapy is reserved for those with life-threatening or enlarging tumors, and in rare occasions, malignant schwannomas. There are no available safety studies with respect to radiotherapy-induced malignant transformation in SWN, though theoretically it is possible given the available data from NF1, and NF2 studies.

Up to date, no clinical trials have been conducted in the setting of SWN and no known effective therapies exist. A case report was published using bevacizumab in one individual with SWN-associated refractory pain with a remarkable response in pain control [115].

6. Clinical trials endpoints in neurofibromatoses

Most early clinical trials for patients with neurofibromatoses used designs and endpoints similar to oncology trials. However, there are major differences in natural history, disease manifestations, and overall prognosis between patients with NF and those with cancers. Hence, there was an unmet need to establish standardized endpoints in NF clinical trials that will allow precise data interpretation and the ability to assess efficacy across different studies. The Response Evaluation in Neurofibromatosis and Schwannomatosis (REiNS) International Collaboration was established in 2011 at the Children's Tumor Foundation (CTF) meeting to achieve consensus about the design for future clinical trials with major emphasis on endpoints. The collaboration included 7 working groups; disease biomarkers; whole-body MRI; functional, visual, patient-reported, and neurocognitive outcome; and imaging for tumor response. Later, two more working groups were added; cutaneous neurofibromas, and patient representation [116].

The REiNS Collaboration published the initial recommendations for clinical trials endpoint in 2013 [117]. MRI with volumetric analysis was recommended as the standard imaging metric for pNF and VS in NF1 and NF2 clinical trials [118]. A 20% volume change was chosen to indicate an increase or decrease in the tumor size. MRI analysis requires central review to ensure consistent results. This is a time and resource intensive tool; thus, the development of methods that can be incorporated into routine clinical practice and can be performed more easily is warranted. Whole-body MRI imaging (WB-MRI) may serve as an endpoint in clinical trials that target multiple tumors. The working group concluded that while WB-MRI is feasible for identifying tumors using both 1.5 T and 3.0 T systems, choosing a standardized image acquisition and analysis methods is crucial for applying WB-MRIs as a tool for assessing tumors in NF [119]. For clinical trials targeting NF2-associated VS, the REiNS functional outcomes group endorsed the use of maximum word recognition score as the primary endpoint for hearing. The group recommended using the measurement of improvement in lip excursion (SMILE) system for studies of facial function [120]. For clinical trials targeting NF-associated OPG, the visual outcomes working group recommended the use of visual acuity as the primary endpoint, as opposed to measurement of tumor size [121]. The group also recommended assessing the optic disc for pallor to allow accurate interpretation of the visual acuity. Regarding the neurocognitive outcomes, the working group concluded that The Digit Span (DS) subtest from the Wechsler scales is the most appropriate performance-based outcome measure, as it provides the best psychometrics, feasibility, and utility across a wide age range, and is extensively used in previous research [122]. For similar reasons, the Conners scale achieved the highest ratings of behavioral questionnaires and is considered the most appropriate observe-rated outcome measure.

It is uncommon for pNF to cause airway compromise or pulmonary dysfunction, yet airway pNFs are clinically important. The REiNS functional outcomes group developed consensus recommendations for sleep and pulmonary outcome endpoints in airway pNFs [123]. The group endorsed using the apnea hypopnea index (AHI) as the primary sleep endpoint, and pulmonary resistance at 10 Hz (R10) of forced expiratory volume in 1 or 0.75 seconds (FEV1 or FEV 0.75) as the primary pulmonary endpoint. The group also identified secondary sleep and pulmonary outcomes. Measures of sleep and pulmonary function may be more clinically meaningful as endpoints than changes in tumor size in clinical trials targeting airway pNFs. Regarding patient-reported outcomes (PRO) of pain and physical function in NF clinical trials, the REiNS working group recommended the numeric rating scale-11 (NRS-11) to assess pain intensity for age 8 years and older [124]. To assess pain interference, the group recommended the Pain Interference Index in pediatric studies and the Patient-Reported Outcome Measurement Information System (PROMIS) Pain Interference Scale in adult studies. PROMIS Physical Function Scale was deemed the most appropriate for NF trials to assess the physical functioning domain. The REiNS disease biomarkers working group reported consensus recommendations to provide clinicians and researches with a common set of guidelines to collect and store biospecimens and for establishment of biobanks for neurofibromatoses [125]. The group described the existing biomarkers in NF and report consensus recommendations for standard operation procedures to standardize sample collection and methodology protocols to promote comparison between studies.

Drug discovery is a very costly and lengthy process, which may take up to 10 years from first-in-human dosing to approval [126]. This process is usually preceded by years of extensive preclinical research to identify suitable targets for clinical development. The REiNS International Collaboration continues to work on developing consensus endpoints in NF clinical trials and to promote early engagement with FDA and other industry partners to accelerate the drug development and approval for NF-associated tumors.

7. Conclusion

The field of NF therapeutics is at inflection point. Several clinical trials have been conducted targeting various manifestations of NF and more studies are ongoing. The alignment of endpoints along with utilizing validated clinical outcomes measures represents a priority for therapeutic development for NF. Fortunately, there is a growing interest in NF, which is drawing the attention of pharmaceutical and biotechnology companies to grow the pipeline for NF targeted therapy. These efforts are combined with several ongoing laboratory and preclinical studies that provide unique opportunities to study the complex biology and natural history of NF-associated tumor. The US breakthrough therapy designation that was granted to Selumetinib in NF1 endorses the critical need for partnership among the major consortia and funders to accelerate the therapeutics development efforts in the NF field.

Disclosures

Mina Lobbous and Bruce Korf report no disclosures relative to the manuscript.

Author details

Mina Lobbous[1*] and Bruce R. Korf[2]

1 Department of Neurology, Division of NeuroOncology, University of Alabama at Birmingham, USA

2 Wayne H. and Sara Crews Finley Endowed Chair in Medical Genetics, University of Alabama at Birmingham, USA

*Address all correspondence to: mlobbous@uabmc.edu

References

[1] Huson SM, Harper PS, Compston DAS. Von recklinghausen neurofibromatosisa clinical and population study in south-east Wales. Brain. 1988;**111**(6):1355-1381. DOI: 10.1093/brain/111.6.1355

[2] Birth incidence and prevalence of tumor-prone syndromes: Estimates from a UK family genetic register service—Evans. American Journal of Medical Genetics Part A—Wiley Online Library. 2010. Available from: https://onlinelibrary.wiley.com/doi/full/10.1002/ajmg.a.33139 [Accessed: 16 June 2019]

[3] Packer RJ et al. Neurofibromatosis clinical trial consortium. Journal of Child Neurology. 2018;**33**(1):82-91. DOI: 10.1177/0883073817739196

[4] Meeting Library. SPRINT: Phase II Study of the MEK 1/2 Inhibitor Selumetinib (AZD6244, ARRY-142886) in Children with Neurofibromatosis Type 1 (NF1) and Inoperable Plexiform Neurofibromas (PN). Available from: https://meetinglibrary.asco.org/record/159508/abstract [Accessed: 24 June 2019]

[5] La Rosa S et al. Delivering on the vision of bench to bedside: A rare disease funding community collaboration to develop effective therapies for neurofibromatosis type 1 tumors. BioRxiv. 2019:552976. DOI: 10.1101/552976

[6] Tucker T, Friedman JM, Friedrich RE, et al. Longitudinal study of neurofibromatosis 1 associated plexiform neurofibromas. Journal of Medical Genetics. 2009;**46**(2):81-85. DOI: 10.1136/jmg.2008.061051

[7] Dombi E, Solomon J, Gillespie AJ, Fox E, Balis FM, Patronas N, et al. NF1 plexiform neurofibroma growth rate by volumetric MRI. Neurology. 2007;**68**(9):643-647. DOI: 10.1212/01.wnl.0000250332.89420.e6

[8] Dombi E, Solomon J, Gillespie AJ, Fox E, Balis FM, et al. NF1 plexiform neurofibroma growth rate by volumetric MRI. Neurology. February 2007;**68**(9):643-647. DOI: 10.1212/01.wnl.0000250332.89420.e6

[9] Prada CE et al. Pediatric plexiform neurofibromas: Impact on morbidity and mortality in neurofibromatosis type 1. The Journal of Pediatrics. 2012;**160**(3):461-467. DOI: 10.1016/j.jpeds.2011.08.051

[10] Widemann BC et al. Phase 2 randomized, flexible crossover, double-blinded, placebo-controlled trial of the farnesyltransferase inhibitor tipifarnib in children and young adults with neurofibromatosis type 1 and progressive plexiform neurofibromas. Neuro-Oncology. 2014;**16**(5):707-718. DOI: 10.1093/neuonc/nou004

[11] Weiss B et al. Sirolimus for progressive neurofibromatosis type 1–associated plexiform neurofibromas: A neurofibromatosis clinical trials consortium phase II study. Neuro-Oncology. 2015;**17**(4):596-603. DOI: 10.1093/neuonc/nou235

[12] Robertson KA, Nalepa G, Yang FC, Bowers DC, Ho CY, Hutchins GD, et al. Imatinib mesylate for plexiform neurofibromas in patients with neurofibromatosis type 1: A phase 2 trial. The Lancet Oncology. 2012;**13**(12):1218-1224. ISSN: 1470-2045. DOI: 10.1016/S1470-2045(12)70414-X

[13] Ratner N, Miller SJ. A RASopathy gene commonly mutated in cancer: The neurofibromatosis type 1 tumour suppressor. Nature Reviews. Cancer. 2015;**15**(5):290-301. DOI: 10.1038/nrc3911

[14] Gupta A et al. Phase I study of thalidomide for the treatment of plexiform neurofibroma in

neurofibromatosis 1. Neurology. 2003;**60**(1):130-132. DOI: 10.1212/01.wnl.0000042321.94839.78

[15] Weiss B, Widemann BC, Wolters P, Dombi E, Vinks A, Cantor A, et al. Sirolimus for progressive neurofibromatosis type 1–associated plexiform neurofibromas: A neurofibromatosis. Clinical Trials Consortium Phase II study. Neuro-Oncology. April 2015;**17**(4):596-603. DOI: 10.1093/neuonc/nou235

[16] Kim AR et al. Phase I trial and pharmacokinetic study of sorafenib in children with neurofibromatosis type I and plexiform neurofibromas. Pediatric Blood & Cancer. 2013;**60**(3):396-401. DOI: 10.1002/pbc.24281

[17] Babovic-Vuksanovic D et al. Phase I trial of pirfenidone in children with neurofibromatosis 1 and plexiform neurofibromas. Pediatric Neurology. 2007;**36**(5):293-300. DOI: 10.1016/j.pediatrneurol.2007.01.009

[18] Widemann BC et al. Phase II trial of pirfenidone in children and young adults with neurofibromatosis type 1 and progressive plexiform neurofibromas. Pediatric Blood & Cancer. 2014;**61**(9):1598-1602. DOI: 10.1002/pbc.25041

[19] Widemann BC, Dombi E, Gillespie A, Wolters PL, Belasco J, Goldman S, et al. Phase 2 randomized, flexible crossover, double-blinded, placebo-controlled trial of the farnesyltransferase inhibitor tipifarnib in children and young adults with neurofibromatosis type 1 and progressive plexiform neurofibromas. Neuro-Oncology. May 2014;**16**(5):707-718. DOI: 10.1093/neuonc/nou004

[20] Phase II trial of pegylated interferon Alfa-2b in young patients with neurofibromatosis type 1 and unresectable plexiform neurofibromas. Neuro-Oncology. Oxford Academic. Available from: https://academic.oup.com/neuro-oncology/article/19/2/289/3038131 [Accessed: 19 June 2019]

[21] Jakacki RI et al. Phase I trial of pegylated interferon-α-2b in young patients with plexiform neurofibromas. Neurology. 2011;**76**(3):265-272. DOI: 10.1212/WNL.0b013e318207b031

[22] Zehou O et al. Absence of efficacy of everolimus in neurofibromatosis 1-related plexiform neurofibromas: Results from a phase 2a trial. Journal of Investigative Dermatology. 2019;**139**(3):718-720. DOI: 10.1016/j.jid.2018.09.016

[23] Robertson KA, Nalepa G, Yang FC, Bowers DC, Ho CY et al. Imatinib mesylate for plexiform neurofibromas in patients with neurofibromatosis type 1: A phase 2 trial. The Lancet Oncology. 2012;**13**(12):1218-1224. ISSN: 1470-2045. DOI: 10.1016/S1470-2045(12)70414-X

[24] Hittson L et al. Phase I study of pexidartinib (PLX3397) in children with refractory leukemias and solid tumors including neurofibromatosis type I (NF1) related plexiform neurofibromas (PN). Journal of Clinical Oncology. 2017;**35**(15_suppl):10546-10546. DOI: 10.1200/JCO.2017.35.15_suppl.10546

[25] Weiss B et al. NFM-06. NF106: Phase 2 trial of the mek inhibitor PD-0325901 in adolescents and adults with nf1-related plexiform neurofibromas: An NF clinical trials consortium study. Neuro-Oncology. 2018;**20**(suppl_2):i143-i143. DOI: 10.1093/neuonc/noy059.514

[26] Dombi E et al. Activity of selumetinib in neurofibromatosis type 1-related plexiform neurofibromas. The New England Journal of Medicine. 2016;**375**(26):2550-2560. DOI: 10.1056/NEJMoa1605943

[27] Lewis RA et al. Von Recklinghausen neurofibromatosis. II. Incidence

of optic gliomata. Ophthalmology. 1984;**91**(8):929-935

[28] Listernick R, Charrow J, Greenwald M, Mets M. Natural history of optic pathway tumors in children with neurofibromatosis type 1: A longitudinal study. The Journal of Pediatrics. 1994;**125**(1):63-66. ISSN: 0022-3476. https://doi.org/10.1016/S0022-3476(94)70122-9

[29] Fisher MJ et al. Visual outcomes in children with neurofibromatosis type 1-associated optic pathway glioma following chemotherapy: A multicenter retrospective analysis. Neuro-Oncology. 2012;**14**(6):790-797. DOI: 10.1093/neuonc/nos076

[30] Packer RJ et al. Carboplatin and vincristine chemotherapy for children with newly diagnosed progressive low-grade gliomas. Journal of Neurosurgery. 1997;**86**(5):747-754. DOI: 10.3171/jns.1997.86.5.0747

[31] Bouffet E et al. Phase II study of weekly vinblastine in recurrent or refractory pediatric low-grade glioma. Journal of Clinical Oncology: Official Journal of the American Society of Clinical Oncology. 2012;**30**(12):1358-1363. DOI: 10.1200/JCO.2011.34.5843

[32] Cappellano AM et al. Single agent vinorelbine in pediatric patients with progressive optic pathway glioma. Journal of Neuro-Oncology. 2015;**121**(2):405-412. DOI: 10.1007/s11060-014-1652-6

[33] Gururangan S et al. Temozolomide in children with progressive low-grade glioma. Neuro-Oncology. 2007;**9**(2):161-168. DOI: 10.1215/15228517-2006-030

[34] Avery RA et al. Marked recovery of vision in children with optic pathway gliomas treated with bevacizumab. JAMA Ophthalmology. 2014;**132**(1):111-114. DOI: 10.1001/jamaophthalmol.2013.5819

[35] Kalin-Hajdu E et al. Visual acuity of children treated with chemotherapy for optic pathway gliomas. Pediatric Blood & Cancer. 2014;**61**(2):223-227. DOI: 10.1002/pbc.24726

[36] Via PD et al. Visual outcome of a cohort of children with neurofibromatosis type 1 and optic pathway glioma followed by a pediatric neuro-oncology program. Neuro-Oncology. 2007;**9**(4):430-437. DOI: 10.1215/15228517-2007-031

[37] Sharif S et al. Second primary tumors in neurofibromatosis 1 patients treated for optic glioma: Substantial risks after radiotherapy. Journal of Clinical Oncology. 2006;**24**(16):2570-2575. DOI: 10.1200/JCO.2005.03.8349

[38] Ullrich NJ et al. Moyamoya following cranial irradiation for primary brain tumors in children. Neurology. 2007;**68**(12):932-938. DOI: 10.1212/01.wnl.0000257095.33125.48

[39] Fangusaro J et al. Selumetinib in paediatric patients with BRAF-aberrant or neurofibromatosis type 1-associated recurrent, refractory, or progressive low-grade glioma: A multicentre, phase 2 trial. The Lancet. Oncology. 2019;**20**(7):1011-1022. DOI: 10.1016/S1470-2045(19)30277-3

[40] Avery RA et al. Handheld optical coherence tomography during sedation in young children with optic pathway gliomas. JAMA Ophthalmology. 2014;**132**(3):265-271. DOI: 10.1001/jamaophthalmol.2013.7649.

[41] Fisher MJ, Avery RA, Allen JC, Ardern-Holmes SL, Bilaniuk LT, Gutmann DH, et al. Functional outcome measures for NF1-associated optic pathway glioma clinical trials. Neurology. For the REiNS International Collaboration. Nov 2013;**81**(21 suppl 1):S15-S24. DOI: 10.1212/01.wnl.0000435745.95155.b88

[42] Abdolrahimzadeh B et al. Neurofibromatosis: An update of ophthalmic characteristics and applications of optical coherence tomography. Clinical Ophthalmology (Auckland, N.Z.). 2016;**10**:851-860. DOI: 10.2147/OPTH.S102830

[43] de Blank P et al. Validation of an automated tractography method for the optic radiations as a biomarker of visual acuity in neurofibromatosis-associated optic pathway glioma. Experimental Neurology, Experimental Approaches to Advance Therapies for Tumors of the Central and Peripheral Nervous System. 2018;**299**:308-316. DOI: 10.1016/j.expneurol.2017.06.004

[44] Rodriguez FJ et al. Gliomas in neurofibromatosis type 1: A clinicopathologic study of 100 patients. Journal of Neuropathology and Experimental Neurology. 2008;**67**(3):240-249. DOI: 10.1097/NEN.0b013e318165eb75

[45] Korf BR. Malignancy in neurofibromatosis type 1. The Oncologist. 2000;**5**(6):477-485. DOI: 10.1634/theoncologist.5-6-477

[46] Huttner AJ et al. Clinicopathologic study of glioblastoma in children with neurofibromatosis type 1. Pediatric Blood & Cancer. 2010;**54**(7):890-896. DOI: 10.1002/pbc.22462

[47] Theeler BJ et al. Prolonged survival in adult neurofibromatosis type I patients with recurrent high-grade gliomas treated with bevacizumab. Journal of Neurology. 2014;**261**(8):1559-1564. DOI: 10.1007/s00415-014-7292-0

[48] D'Angelo F et al. The molecular landscape of glioma in patients with neurofibromatosis 1. Nature Medicine. 2019;**25**(1):176-187. DOI: 10.1038/s41591-018-0263-8

[49] Ducatman BS et al. Malignant peripheral nerve sheath tumors. A clinicopathologic study of 120 cases. Cancer. 1986;**57**(10):2006-2021. DOI: 10.1002/1097-0142(19860515)57:10<2006::aid-cncr2820571022>3.0.co;2-6

[50] Evans D et al. Malignant peripheral nerve sheath tumours in neurofibromatosis 1. Journal of Medical Genetics. 2002;**39**(5):311-314. DOI: 10.1136/jmg.39.5.311

[51] Watson MA et al. Gene expression profiling reveals unique molecular subtypes of neurofibromatosis type I-associated and sporadic malignant peripheral nerve sheath tumors. Brain Pathology. 2004;**14**(3):297-303. DOI: 10.1111/j.1750-3639.2004.tb00067.x

[52] Brekke HR et al. Genomic changes in chromosomes 10, 16, and X in malignant peripheral nerve sheath tumors identify a high-risk patient group. Journal of Clinical Oncology. 2010;**28**(9):1573-1582. DOI: 10.1200/JCO.2009.24.8989

[53] Bredella MA et al. Value of PET in the assessment of patients with neurofibromatosis type 1. American Journal of Roentgenology. 2007;**189**(4):928-935. DOI: 10.2214/AJR.07.2060

[54] Ferner RE et al. [18F]2-fluoro-2-deoxy-D-glucose positron emission tomography (FDG PET) as a diagnostic tool for Neurofibromatosis 1 (NF1) associated malignant peripheral nerve sheath tumours (MPNSTs): A long-term clinical study. Annals of Oncology. 2008;**19**(2):390-394. DOI: 10.1093/annonc/mdm450

[55] Meany H, Widemann BC, Ratner N. Malignant peripheral nerve sheath tumors: Prognostic and diagnostic markers and therapeutic targets. Neurofibromatosis Type 1: Molecular and Cellular Biology. 2012;**2**:445-467. DOI: 10.1007/978-3-642-32864-0_29

[56] Kahn J, Gillespie A, Tsokos M, Ondos J, Dombi E, Camphausen K, et al. Radiation therapy in management of sporadic and neurofibromatosis type 1-associated malignant peripheral nerve sheath tumors. Frontiers in Oncology. 2014;**4**:324. DOI: 10.3389/fonc.2014.00324

[57] Santoro A et al. Doxorubicin versus CYVADIC versus doxorubicin plus ifosfamide in first-line treatment of advanced soft tissue sarcomas: A randomized study of the european organization for research and treatment of cancer soft tissue and bone sarcoma group. Journal of Clinical Oncology: Official Journal of the American Society of Clinical Oncology. 1995;**13**(7):1537-1545. DOI: 10.1200/JCO.1995.13.7.1537

[58] Kroep JR et al. First-line chemotherapy for malignant peripheral nerve sheath tumor (MPNST) versus other histological soft tissue sarcoma subtypes and as a prognostic factor for MPNST: An EORTC soft tissue and bone sarcoma group study. Annals of Oncology. 2011;**22**(1):207-214. DOI: 10.1093/annonc/mdq338

[59] Widemann BC et al. SARC016: Phase II study of everolimus in combination with bevacizumab in sporadic and neurofibromatosis type 1 (NF1) related refractory malignant peripheral nerve sheath tumors (MPNST). Journal of Clinical Oncology. 2016;**34**(15_suppl):11053-11053. DOI: 10.1200/JCO.2016.34.15_suppl.11053

[60] Epidermal Growth Factor Receptor Signaling Pathways Are Associated with Tumorigenesis in the Nf1:P53 Mouse Tumor Model. Cancer Research. Available from: http://cancerres.aacrjournals.org/content/62/15/4507.short [Accessed: 21 June 2019]

[61] Chugh R et al. Phase II multicenter trial of Imatinib in 10 histologic subtypes of sarcoma using a Bayesian hierarchical statistical model. Journal of Clinical Oncology. 2009;**27**(19):3148-3153. DOI: 10.1200/JCO.2008.20.5054

[62] Results of a Sarcoma Alliance for Research through Collaboration (SARC) Phase II Trial of Dasatinib in Previously Treated, High-grade, advanced sarcoma. Journal of Clinical Oncology. Available from: https://ascopubs.org/doi/abs/10.1200/jco.2010.28.15_suppl.10009 [Accessed: 21 June 2019]

[63] Maki RG et al. Phase II study of sorafenib in patients with metastatic or recurrent sarcomas. Journal of Clinical Oncology. 2009;**27**(19):3133-3140. DOI: 10.1200/JCO.2008.20.4495

[64] Phase II Study of Erlotinib in Metastatic or Unresectable Malignant Peripheral Nerve Sheath Tumors (MPNST). Journal of Clinical Oncology. Available from: https://ascopubs.org/doi/abs/10.1200/jco.2006.24.18_suppl.9518 [Accessed: 21 June 2019]

[65] Vogel KS et al. Mouse tumor model for neurofibromatosis type 1. Science. 1999;**286**(5447);2176-2179. DOI: 10.1126/science.286.5447.2176

[66] Cichowski K et al. Mouse models of tumor development in neurofibromatosis type 1. Science. 1999;**286**(5447):2172-2176. DOI: 10.1126/science.286.5447.2172

[67] Johansson G et al. Effective in vivo targeting of the mammalian target of rapamycin pathway in malignant peripheral nerve sheath tumors. Molecular Cancer Therapeutics. 2008;**7**(5):1237-1245. DOI: 10.1158/1535-7163.MCT-07-2335

[68] De Raedt T et al. Exploiting cancer cell vulnerabilities to develop a combination therapy for Ras-driven tumors. Cancer Cell. 2011;**20**(3):400-413. DOI: 10.1016/j.ccr.2011.08.014

[69] Kim AR et al. SARC023: Phase I/II trial of ganetespib in combination with sirolimus for refractory sarcomas and malignant peripheral nerve sheath tumors (MPNST). Journal of Clinical Oncology. 2014;**32**(15_suppl):TPS10603. DOI: 10.1200/jco.2014.32.15_suppl.tps10603

[70] Deyle DR et al. Oncolytic measles virus as a novel therapy for malignant peripheral nerve sheath tumors. Gene. 2015;**565**(1):140-145. DOI: 10.1016/j.gene.2015.04.001

[71] Ferner RE et al. Guidelines for the diagnosis and management of individuals with neurofibromatosis 1. Journal of Medical Genetics. 2006;**44**(2):81-88. DOI: 10.1136/jmg.2006.045906

[72] Page PZ et al. Impact of neurofibromatosis 1 on quality of life: A cross-sectional study of 176 American cases. American Journal of Medical Genetics Part A. 2006;**140A**(18):1893-1898. DOI: 10.1002/ajmg.a.31422

[73] Lutterodt CG, Mohan A, Kirkpatrick N. The use of electrodessication in the treatment of cutaneous neurofibromatosis: A retrospective patient satisfaction outcome assessment. Journal of Plastic, Reconstructive & Aesthetic Surgery. 2016;**69**(6):765-769. DOI: 10.1016/j.bjps.2016.03.024

[74] Méni C, Sbidian E, Moreno JC, Lafaye S, Buffard V, Wolkenstein P, et al. Treatment of Neurofibromas with a Carbon Dioxide Laser: A Retrospective Cross-Sectional Study of 106 Patients. Dermatology. 2015;**230**:263-268. DOI: 10.1159/000368078

[75] Elwakil TF, Samy NA, Elbasiouny MS. Non-excision treatment of multiple cutaneous neurofibromas by laser photocoagulation. Lasers in Medical Science. 2008;**23**(3):301-306. DOI: 10.1007/s10103-007-0485-3

[76] Kim S-H et al. Radiofrequency ablation and excision of multiple cutaneous lesions in neurofibromatosis type 1. Archives of Plastic Surgery. 2013;**40**(1):57-61. DOI: 10.5999/aps.2013.40.1.57

[77] Dolmans DEJGJ, Fukumura D, Jain RK. Photodynamic therapy for cancer. Nature Reviews Cancer. 2003;**3**(5):380. DOI: 10.1038/nrc1071

[78] Riccardi VM. Ketotifen suppression of NF1 neurofibroma growth over 30 years. American Journal of Medical Genetics Part A. 2015;**167**(7):1570-1577. DOI: 10.1002/ajmg.a.37045

[79] Koenig MK et al. Topical rapamycin therapy to alleviate the cutaneous manifestations of tuberous sclerosis complex. Drugs in R&D. 2012;**12**(3):121-126. DOI: 10.2165/11634580-000000000-00000

[80] Verma SK et al. Considerations for development of therapies for cutaneous neurofibroma. Neurology. 2018;**91**(2 Suppl 1):S21-S30. DOI: 10.1212/WNL.0000000000005791

[81] Slopis JM et al. Treatment of disfiguring cutaneous lesions in neurofibromatosis-1 with everolimus: A phase II, open-label, single-arm trial. Drugs in R&D. 2018;**18**(4):295-302. DOI: 10.1007/s40268-018-0248-6

[82] Cannon A et al. Clinical trial design for cutaneous neurofibromas. Neurology. 2018;**91**(2 Suppl 1): S31-S37. DOI: 10.1212/WNL.0000000000005790

[83] Evans D et al. Incidence of vestibular schwannoma and neurofibromatosis 2 in the north west of England over a 10-year period: Higher incidence than previously thought. Otology & Neurotology. 2005;**26**(1):93-97

[84] Gutmann DH et al. The diagnostic evaluation and multidisciplinary

management of neurofibromatosis 1 and neurofibromatosis 2. JAMA. 1997;**278**(1):51-57. DOI: 10.1001/jama.1997.03550010065042

[85] Fisher LM et al. Concordance of bilateral vestibular schwannoma growth and hearing changes in neurofibromatosis 2: Neurofibromatosis 2 natural history consortium. Otology & Neurotology. 2009;**30**(6):835. DOI: 10.1097/MAO.0b013e3181b2364c

[86] Otsuka G et al. Age at symptom onset and long-term survival in patients with neurofibromatosis type 2. Journal of Neurosurgery. 2003;**99**(3):480-483. DOI: 10.3171/jns.2003.99.3.0480

[87] Choi JW et al. Clinical course of vestibular schwannoma in pediatric neurofibromatosis type 2: Clinical article. Journal of Neurosurgery: Pediatrics. 2014;**13**(6):650-657. DOI: 10.3171/2014.3.PEDS13455

[88] Goutagny S, Kalamarides M. Meningiomas and neurofibromatosis. Journal of Neuro-Oncology. 2010;**99**(3):341-347. DOI: 10.1007/s11060-010-0339-x

[89] Wilding A et al. Life expectancy in hereditary cancer predisposing diseases: An observational study. Journal of Medical Genetics. 2012;**49**(4):264-269. DOI: 10.1136/jmedgenet-2011-100562

[90] Hanemann CO. Magic but treatable? Tumours due to loss of Merlin. Brain. 2008;**131**(3):606-615. DOI: 10.1093/brain/awm249

[91] Tos M et al. What is the real incidence of vestibular schwannoma? Archives of Otolaryngology—Head & Neck Surgery. 2004;**130**(2):216-220. DOI: 10.1001/archotol.130.2.216

[92] Combs SE et al. Long-term outcome of stereotactic radiosurgery (SRS) in patients with acoustic neuromas. International Journal of Radiation Oncology*Biology*Physics. 2006;**64**(5):1341-1347. DOI: 10.1016/j.ijrobp.2005.10.024

[93] Choi et al. Clinical Course of Vestibular Schwannoma in Pediatric Neurofibromatosis Type 2

[94] Evans DGR et al. Management of the patient and family with neurofibromatosis 2: A consensus conference statement. British Journal of Neurosurgery. 2005;**19**(1):5-12. DOI: 10.1080/02688690500081206

[95] Neurofibromatosis 2, radiosurgery and malignant nervous system tumours. British Journal of Cancer. 2000;**82**(4):998. DOI: 10.1054/bjoc.1999.1030

[96] III Slattery WH et al. Vestibular schwannoma growth rates in neurofibromatosis type 2 natural history consortium subjects. Otology & Neurotology. 2004;**25**(5):811

[97] Plotkin SR et al. Natural history of vestibular schwannoma growth and hearing decline in newly diagnosed neurofibromatosis type 2 patients. Otology & Neurotology. 2014;**35**(1):e50. DOI: 10.1097/MAO.0000000000000239

[98] Peyre M et al. Conservative management of bilateral vestibular schwannomas in neurofibromatosis type 2 patients: Hearing and tumor growth results. Neurosurgery. 2013;**72**(6):907-914. DOI: 10.1227/NEU.0b013e31828bae28

[99] Gareth Evans D et al. Consensus recommendations to accelerate clinical trials for neurofibromatosis type 2. Clinical Cancer Research. 2009;**15**(16):5032-5039. DOI: 10.1158/1078-0432.CCR-08-3011

[100] Plotkin SR et al. Bevacizumab for progressive vestibular schwannoma in neurofibromatosis

type 2: A retrospective review of 31 patients. Otology & Neurotology. 2012;**33**(6):1046. DOI: 10.1097/MAO.0b013e31825e73f5

[101] Plotkin SR et al. Hearing improvement after bevacizumab in patients with neurofibromatosis type 2. New England Journal of Medicine. 2009;**361**(4):358-367. DOI: 10.1056/NEJMoa0902579

[102] Plotkin SR, Tonsgard JH, Ullrich NJ, Allen JC, Rosser TL, et al. Preliminary report of a multicenter, phase 2 study of bevacizumab in children and adults with neurofibromatosis 2 and progressive vestibular schwannomas: An NF clinical trials consortium study. Journal of Clinical Oncology. 2018;**36**(15_suppl):2056-2056. DOI: 10.1200/JCO.2018.36.15_suppl.2056

[103] Troutman S et al. Crizotinib inhibits NF2-associated schwannoma through inhibition of focal adhesion kinase 1. Oncotarget. 2016;7(34):54515-54525. DOI: 10.18632/oncotarget.10248

[104] Karajannis MA et al. Phase II study of everolimus in children and adults with neurofibromatosis type 2 and progressive vestibular schwannomas. Neuro-Oncology. 2014;**16**(2):292-297. DOI: 10.1093/neuonc/not150

[105] Goutagny S et al. Phase II study of MTORC1 inhibition by everolimus in neurofibromatosis type 2 patients with growing vestibular schwannomas. Journal of Neuro-Oncology. 2015;**122**(2):313-320. DOI: 10.1007/s11060-014-1710-0

[106] Karajannis MA et al. Phase II trial of lapatinib in adult and pediatric patients with neurofibromatosis type 2 and progressive vestibular schwannomas. Neuro-Oncology. 2012;**14**(9):1163-1170. DOI: 10.1093/neuonc/nos146

[107] Blakeley JO et al. Efficacy and biomarker study of bevacizumab for hearing loss resulting from neurofibromatosis type 2-associated vestibular schwannomas. Journal of Clinical Oncology: Official Journal of the American Society of Clinical Oncology. 2016;**34**(14):1669-1675. DOI: 10.1200/JCO.2015.64.3817

[108] Hans VH. Schwannomatosis. Neurology. 2009;**72**(13):1188-1189. DOI: 10.1212/01.wnl.0000339391.48966.ab

[109] Merker V et al. Clinical features of the schwannomatosis tumor suppressor syndrome: A retrospective analysis of 87 patients (S45.003). Neurology. 2012;**78**(1 Supplement):S45.003

[110] Plotkin SR et al. Update from the 2011 international Schwannomatosis workshop: From genetics to diagnostic criteria. American Journal of Medical Genetics Part A. 2013;**161**(3):405-416. DOI: 10.1002/ajmg.a.35760

[111] Smith MJ et al. SMARCB1 mutations in Schwannomatosis and genotype correlations with rhabdoid tumors. Cancer Genetics. 2014;**207**(9):373-378. DOI: 10.1016/j.cancergen.2014.04.001

[112] Piotrowski A et al. Germline loss-of-function mutations in LZTR1 predispose to an inherited disorder of multiple schwannomas. Nature Genetics. 2014;**46**(2):182-187. DOI: 10.1038/ng.2855

[113] MacCollin M, Chiocca EA, Evans DG, Friedman JM, Horvitz R, Jaramillo M, et al. Diagnostic criteria for schwannomatosis. Neurology. Jun 2005;**64**(11):1838-1845. DOI: 10.1212/01. WNL.0000163982.78900. AD

[114] Merker VL, Esparza S, Smith MJ, Stemmer-Rachamimov A, Plotkin SR. Clinical features of schwannomatosis: A Retrospective analysis of 87 patients.

The Oncologist. 2012;**17**:1317-1322. First published on August 27, 2012. DOI: 10.1634/theoncologist.2012-0162

[115] Blakeley J et al. Clinical response to bevacizumab in schwannomatosis. Neurology. 2014;**83**(21):1986. DOI: 10.1212/WNL.0000000000000997

[116] Plotkin SR et al. Achieving consensus for clinical trials: The REiNS international collaboration. Neurology. 2013;**81**(21 suppl 1): S1-S5. DOI: 10.1212/01.wnl.0000435743.49414.b6

[117] Widemann BC et al. Conclusions and future directions for the REiNS international collaboration. Neurology. 2013;**81**(21 suppl 1):S41. DOI: 10.1212/01.wnl.0000435748.79908.c5

[118] Dombi E et al. Recommendations for imaging tumor response in neurofibromatosis clinical trials. Neurology. 2013;**81**(21 suppl 1): S33-S40. DOI: 10.1212/01.wnl.0000435744.57038.af

[119] Ahlawat S et al. Current whole-body MRI applications in the neurofibromatoses. Neurology. 2016;**87**(7 Suppl 1):S31-S39. DOI: 10.1212/WNL.0000000000002929

[120] Plotkin SR et al. Hearing and facial function outcomes for neurofibromatosis 2 clinical trials. Neurology. 2013;**81**(21 suppl 1):S25. DOI: 10.1212/01.wnl.0000435746.02780.f6

[121] Fisher MJ, Avery RA, Allen JC, Ardern-Holmes SL, Bilaniuk LT et al. Functional outcome measures for NF1-associated optic pathway glioma clinical trials. Neurology. For the REiNS International Collaboration. Nov 2013;**81**(21 suppl 1):S15-S24. DOI: 10.1212/01.wnl.0000435745.95155.b8

[122] Walsh KS et al. Neurocognitive outcomes in neurofibromatosis clinical trials. Neurology. 2016;**87**(7 Suppl 1):S21-S30. DOI: 10.1212/WNL.0000000000002928

[123] Plotkin SR et al. Sleep and pulmonary outcomes for clinical trials of airway plexiform neurofibromas in NF1. Neurology. 2016;**87** (7 Suppl 1):S13-S20. DOI: 10.1212/WNL.0000000000002933

[124] Wolters PL et al. Patient-reported outcomes of pain and physical functioning in neurofibromatosis clinical trials. Neurology. 2016;**87**(7 Suppl 1):S4-S12. DOI: 10.1212/WNL.0000000000002927

[125] Oliver Hanemann C et al. Current status and recommendations for biomarkers and biobanking in neurofibromatosis. Neurology. 2016;**87**(7 Suppl 1):S40-S48. DOI: 10.1212/WNL.0000000000002932

[126] Hay M et al. Clinical development success rates for investigational drugs. Nature Biotechnology. 2014;**32**:40-51. DOI: 10.1038/nbt.2786